# MAKING A MEDIC

# MAKING A MEDIC

## The Ultimate Guide to Medical School

### DAVID BRILL

MBBS, BSc Neuroscience, MSc Science Communication

Foundation trainee doctor
Royal Free London NHS Foundation Trust

Scion

ISBN 9781911510444

First published 2019

A CIP catalogue record for this book is available from the British Library.

**Scion Publishing Limited**

The Old Hayloft, Vantage Business Park, Bloxham Road, Banbury OX16 9UX, UK
www.scionpublishing.com

**Important Note from the Publisher**

**Our medical textbooks are assessed and reviewed by the following medical students:**

| | | |
|---|---|---|
| Nora Aljamil | Umar Dinah | Marco Narajas |
| Adam Arshad | Keziah Element | Toby Nicholls |
| Tanith Bain | Sophie Gunter | Simran Piya |
| Susan Baird | Laura Hartley | Ross Porter |
| Nabeela Bhaloo | Zoe Johnson | Macauley Shaw |
| Amy Campbell | Victoria Kinkaid | Jay Singh |
| Thomas Charles | Dylan McClurg | Paris Tatt-Smith |
| Jason Cheong Kah Chun | Connor McKee | Bhavesh Tailor |
| Yasmine Cherfi | Kate McMurrugh | Charlotte Thompson |
| Amaan Din | Jonathan Mok | Jack Whiting |

We are grateful for their essential feedback. If you would like to apply to be a student reviewer, please contact **simon.watkins@scionpublishing.com** in the first instance.

Cover design by Andrew Magee Design Ltd
Typeset by Evolution Design & Digital Ltd (Kent)
Printed in the UK

Last digit is the print number: 10 9 8 7 6 5 4 3 2 1

# Contents

## Chapter 1 Golden rules for surviving medical school

## Chapter 2 Preclinical years

## Chapter 3 Your first clinical year

## Chapter 4 Second clinical year

## Chapter 5 Final year

# Foreword

New medical students have always gained much from the experiences of peers ahead of them. *Making a Medic* offers such support from David Brill, an exemplary graduate of St George's, by describing the myriad successful and innovative learning strategies that he employed to navigate the intensity of a medical course, including for example: his search for the depth and breadth of knowledge needed for safe passage through exams and onward travel to excellent clinical practice, and the identification of high value clinical exposures to make learning efficient. David does this by taking the reader on an affirmative journey from medical school entry to Foundation application, offering his diverse learning techniques for the knowledge-dense years of clinical science, the academic, practical and emotional challenges of clinical placements, and the navigation of assessments, career choices and electives. For the educational milieu of each phase, the book presents nuanced content on how to actively and efficiently learn, retain enthusiasm for learning, and continue to enjoy medicine. Coming from a doctor with a professional science writing background, it is no surprise to find that it is very well written and enjoyable to read. The fun and clear diagrams add texture. It's one of those books that students will benefit from reading as soon as they start medical school and will then return to each time their learning environment changes. I don't know how David had time to write this during FY1, but many students will be very glad that he did.

*Dr Judith Ibison*
*Reader in Primary Care*
*St George's, University of London*

# Preface

If you've picked up *Making a Medic*, you're presumably at medical school, about to start medical school or just considering applying. Whatever the case, welcome, and well done for taking the first steps towards an exciting, varied and immensely challenging career. I hope this book will help make your studies as enjoyable, rewarding and pain free as possible.

*Chapter 1* applies to all of medical school and can be read at any time. However, to get the most out of the book, I'd suggest you only read the other chapters at the beginning of the year/years they apply to and then return to them throughout that year. For example, you should read *Chapter 2* at the beginning of your preclinical years and then keep coming back to it as and when you need. Then read *Chapter 3* at the start of your first clinical year, and so on. This approach will help keep things relevant to your stage of training and avoid overloading you with too much information too early. But, if you do want to read the whole book in one go, then of course you are welcome to do so!

Studying medicine is an intensely personal experience – there is no single way to go about it – and there is enormous variation between medical schools. Not everything I have suggested in this book will work for everyone at every stage of every medical school. That's absolutely fine! My intention is for you to pick and choose the bits that work for you and to dip in and out as you progress through your degree, not to slavishly follow the entire script in order. Ultimately you will need to find your own path: my advice is just intended to guide you towards it.

Why did I write this book? I forget exactly when and where the idea came to me, but it was probably whilst aimlessly traipsing around a hospital ward absent-mindedly wondering whether it was urine, faeces or both that I could smell. Or the patients' lunches being warmed up. It was not a sudden brainwave; more the gradual realisation that I was not the first medical student to be bored to tears on a clinical placement, learning nothing and feeling useless and frustrated. In fact, there had been countless thousands of students before me, all traipsing the same corridors, feeling the same emotions and asking themselves the same questions: am I wasting my time? How can I get more out of my placements? How much of this stuff do I *actually* need to know? Can they really expect us to learn *all of medicine* in just a few years?

The answers to these questions, I soon discovered, come from students in the years above. They've already been there, seen it, done it and passed the exams to prove it. They're full of useful tips about how to study, which resources to use, how to get the most out of placements and how to ace your OSCEs. They're regular human beings like you and me, and the vast majority survive medical school, go on to pass finals and become doctors. They are living proof that, no matter how long and hard this degree may seem, everything will be okay in the end.

The more I thought about it, the more surprised I became that hardly any of this wisdom had been written down. There were entire libraries full of scientific and clinical information, but barely any advice on how to use it sensibly whilst keeping your sanity intact. And so somewhere in my penultimate year, I began jotting down ideas: things I wished I'd known when I started medical school, things I had done well over the years and things I felt I could have done better. These notes expanded into a complete guide covering everything you need to know to survive as a modern-day medical student, and *Making a Medic* was born.

Why should you bother listening to me? Well, for starters, I'm not an academic in an ivory tower: I have just been there and done it myself, it's fresh in my mind and I know what it takes to succeed without going insane in the process. I aced medical school not because I was the best or brightest student in the year (I wasn't), or had the most free time to study (I **definitely** didn't), but because I studied effectively, efficiently and had excellent coping strategies. I worked my nuts off, I won't lie to you, but I did so in a realistic, sustainable way that allowed me to maintain a healthy work–life balance. I play a lot of sport, have a good social life and am happily married with three young children. And crucially, having avoided burnout at medical school, I am actually enjoying life as an FY1 and remain excited and enthusiastic about medicine. You might be at a very different age and stage of life to me, but my strategies and ideas are universally applicable and it can only help you to take them on board!

Medical school is many things to many people: it can bring joy, pain, laughter, tears and many more emotions besides. In the end, it's what you make of it, and I hope your experience will be as positive and rewarding as mine. It won't always be easy, but nothing that's truly worth doing ever is. I hope that in some small measure, *Making a Medic* will support and help you along the way.

*David Brill*

# Acknowledgements

Special thanks to all my fellow George's students for sharing an often mad, occasionally absurd, but immensely enjoyable four years of my life. In particular, Dan, Joe, James, Tim, Karen and the three Hannahs, without whom my study groups and mock OSCEs would have been $n = 1$. Thanks also to the many amazing teachers, supervisors and colleagues who supported me along the way, to my fellow FY1s at Barnet for all their helpful suggestions, and to the team at Scion for taking a punt on me and my idea and turning it into reality. Mum, Dad, Rick, Lisa, Simon, Anna, Tessa and Fergal: you have helped and supported me in more ways than I can even begin to count, and I appreciate it all. Sylvie, Ted and Raya: I'm glad you like my cartoons. Now please stop asking me to read this book to you as a bedtime story because it just isn't going to work. And finally: to Eve, without whom absolutely none of this would have been possible. You encouraged me to apply to medical school, stuck with me through the many highs and lows and are miraculously still there for me on the other side. You've made this book better and you've made me better. Thank you.

# Abbreviations

| | |
|---|---|
| A&E | accident & emergency |
| ABG | arterial blood gas |
| ACE | angiotensin-converting enzyme |
| ACS | acute coronary syndrome |
| AKI | acute kidney injury |
| AP | anteroposterior |
| BMA | British Medical Association |
| BMAT | Biomedical Admissions Test |
| BNF / BNFc | British National Formulary / for children |
| BNP | B-type natriuretic peptide |
| BTS | British Thoracic Society |
| CBD | case-based discussion |
| CEX | clinical evaluation exercise (often called mini-CEX) |
| COPD | chronic obstructive pulmonary disease |
| COW | computer on wheels |
| CPH/PPD | community and population health / personal and professional development |
| CRP | C-reactive protein |
| CT | computed tomography |
| CTPA | CT pulmonary angiogram |
| CXR | chest X-ray |
| DNAR | do not attempt resuscitation |
| DOP | directly observed procedure |
| DVT | deep vein thrombosis |
| ECG | electrocardiogram |
| ENT | ear, nose and throat |
| EPM | educational performance measure |
| ERCP | endoscopic retrograde cholangiopancreatography |
| FBC | full blood count |
| FOMO | fear of missing out |
| FY | foundation year |
| GAMSAT | Graduate Medical School Admissions Test |
| GI | gastrointestinal |
| GMC | General Medical Council |
| GORD | gastro-oesophageal reflux disease |
| GP | general practitioner |
| GTN | glyceryl trinitrate |
| HbA1C | glycosylated haemoglobin |
| HIV | human immunodeficiency virus |
| HLA | human leukocyte antigen |
| ICD | implantable cardioverter defibrillator |
| ICE | ideas, concerns and expectations |
| IV | intravenous |
| JVP | jugular venous pressure |
| LABA | long-acting beta agonist |
| LFTs | liver function tests |
| LOBs | learning objectives |
| LVH | left ventricular hypertrophy |
| MCQ | multiple choice question |
| MDT | multidisciplinary team |
| MHC | major histocompatibility complex |
| NAI | non-accidental injury |
| NHS | National Health Service |
| NICE | National Institute for Health and Care Excellence |
| NSAIDs | non-steroidal anti-inflammatory drugs |
| NSTEMI | non-ST-elevation myocardial infarction |
| O&G | obstetrics and gynaecology |
| Obs | a patient's observations, aka vital signs |
| OCD | obsessive–compulsive disorder |
| OD | once daily |
| ODP | operating department practitioner |

| | | | |
|---|---|---|---|
| OSCE | Objective Structured Clinical Exam | SSC / SSM | student-selected component / module |
| PA | posteroanterior | SSRIs | selective serotonin reuptake inhibitors |
| PBL | problem-based learning | | |
| PC | presenting complaint | STEMI | ST-elevation myocardial infarction |
| PCI | percutaneous coronary intervention | STI | sexually transmitted infection |
| PDA | patent ductus arteriosus | T3 / T4 | triiodothyronine / thyroxine |
| PEF / PEFR | peak expiratory flow / rate | TFTs | thyroid function tests |
| PPI | proton pump inhibitor | TIA | transient ischaemic attack |
| PR | per rectum | TOF | trans-oesophageal fistula |
| PRN | as required (from the Latin *pro re nata*) | TRH | thyrotropin-releasing hormone |
| | | TSH | thyroid-stimulating hormone |
| PSA | Prescribing Safety Assessment | TTA / TTO | to take away / out |
| QIP | quality improvement project | U&Es | urea and electrolytes |
| SABA | short-acting beta agonist | UCAT | University Clinical Aptitude Test (previously known as UKCAT) |
| SDL | self-directed learning | | |
| SHO | senior house officer | UKMLA | UK Medical Licensing Assessment |
| SIADH | syndrome of inappropriate antidiuretic hormone secretion | UoA | unit of application, aka deanery |
| | | UTI | urinary tract infection |
| SIGN | Scottish Intercollegiate Guidelines Network | VSD | ventricular septal defect |
| | | VTE | venous thromboembolism |
| SJT | Situational Judgement Test | WHO | World Health Organisation |

# Chapter 1
# Golden rules for surviving medical school

## Contents

# 1.1 Look after yourself

Before you read another word, put this book down for a minute and go look in the mirror. The person staring back at you has achieved something absolutely amazing by getting into medical school. You've run the gauntlet of A levels, personal statements, interviews and work experience. You've passed the BMAT, GAMSAT or UCAT, done all the paperwork and convinced the right people that you have what it takes to become a doctor. You probably spent a lot of money and got very stressed along the way but never mind that now because **you did it**! You're one of 7500 new medical students to make the cut from 21000 applicants, not to mention the countless thousands who didn't even bother to apply. Pat yourself on the back, because you have every right to feel extremely proud of yourself.

Never forget this feeling, no matter what the next few years throw at you. Medical school can be an incredible, rewarding and life-changing experience, but it can also be a long, demanding and stressful road riddled with challenging twists and turns. I don't wish to sound bleak but it would be remiss of me not to warn you that there may be hard times ahead. The statistics, sadly, bear this out, with around 27% of medical students reporting depressive symptoms, higher than the general population.[1] It's important to enter with your eyes open to these facts, so you can put strategies in place to protect yourself from day one.

**Absolutely none of it is worthwhile if it costs your mental or physical health in the process. Your wellbeing must always take priority over studies, exams and placements, no matter what.**

At my graduation, one speaker asked us to stand up and applaud our friends, family and loved ones who had supported us through medical school. I will always remember that, because he hit the nail on the head: even if you don't realise it yet, you are going to rely heavily on those around you for emotional, spiritual, financial and academic support to survive medical school. This is perhaps the single best thing you can do to look after yourself: make sure you have a strong network in place whom you can talk to, trust and rely upon. Appreciate them, love them and remember they are there for you when things get tough. I know I couldn't have done it without them.

---

1 *BMJ* 2017;357:j1460

**Six ways to preserve your sanity at medical school:**
1.  Have realistic expectations: medical school is going to be long and difficult.
2.  Be proud of yourself and what you have already achieved.
3.  Make time for yourself in amongst all the studying.
4.  Maintain a life and activities away from medicine and medical people.
5.  Talk openly to your friends, family or a professional if you are struggling.
6.  Keep things in perspective: no degree is worth ruining your life over.

You should also familiarise yourself with your medical school's support services and know who you can reach out to. This will probably be covered in freshers' week when you are on an excited high and feel this information doesn't apply to you, but listen up because you never know when you might need it. There is a lot happening at a national level too: the BMA has some great online resources and a 24/7 confidential counselling service (call 0330 123 1245), while the GMC is working with medical schools to try to increase the amount of support available.[2,3] Also ensure you register with a local GP – it's astonishing how many medical students don't do this – and never be afraid to seek their help when you need it. The Samaritans are there 24/7 (call 116 123), along with PAPYRUS HOPELINEUK for under-35s from 10 a.m. to 10 p.m. (call 0800 068 4141 or text 07786 209 697). Whatever happens, know that you are not alone.

If you are ever feeling out of your depth at medical school, which I did *a lot* of the time, it's probably because you're looking up at the people above you in the medical food chain and thinking how far you still have to go. Instead, take a minute to look sideways and down and appreciate how far you have already come. That begins with remembering that proud face in the mirror: you have done brilliantly to get in, you deserve to be there and you 100% have what it takes to succeed. Never let anyone tell you otherwise!

# 1.2 Embrace variety

Day one of medical school. You've waved goodbye to your parents, moved into halls of residence and met the people you're going to spend the next few years of your life with. Your loan is sorted, you've Instagrammed your

2 www.bma.org.uk/advice/work-life-support/your-wellbeing
3 www.gmc-uk.org/education/standards-guidance-and-curricula/guidance/supporting-medical-students-with-mental-health-conditions

new stethoscope and piled a bunch of serious-looking textbooks onto your desk. What else can you can do to ensure you get off to the best possible start at medical school?

Perhaps the most important thing, in my view, is to put yourself in the right mindset to survive the next 4–6 years of intensive learning without your brain exploding in a mushroom cloud of squidgy goop. And the key to this is to embrace **variety** – to realise that there is no single method or style for studying medicine, but rather an infinite range of learning opportunities which you will need to grab hold of. To maximise these, you must make yourself a flexible learner who can extract the most from any situation, whether it's a lecture from an esteemed professor or study time alone in the library, attending an antenatal clinic, or visiting a high-security psychiatric hospital. Nor should you limit yourself to particular study techniques or resources: be prepared to use print **and** electronic, pictures **and** text; to study alone **and** in groups.

I say this because there is loads of literature out there encouraging you to figure out your 'learning style' and stick to it. You're either a visual or an auditory learner; or perhaps a kinaesthetic or logical learner, depending which model you choose to follow. But this makes little sense to me: why do you need to pigeon-hole yourself in this way? Why can't you be different things at different times, or everything all at once? Medicine is one of the broadest and most diverse subjects on earth: in my view it's unhelpful to set narrow limits on the way you approach it. I did extremely well without ever labelling myself like this! I drew pictures, watched videos, listened to podcasts **and** wrote notes. I used my eyes, my ears, my hands, my head **and** my heart. I solved some problems through logic; others through instinct and countless more by plain old guesswork. I don't know what style of learner that makes me and frankly I don't really care!

**TOP TIPS:**

- Don't pigeon-hole your 'learning style' or restrict yourself to certain techniques.
- Try anything and everything to begin with, and keep using different techniques for different subjects. Take your time discovering what works best for you and grab any opportunity that comes your way.

I will expand later on all these different learning opportunities, but adopt this mantra from day one: *I am a flexible learner. Variety is my friend.* Not only will this keep your mind fresh and help avoid boredom, but it will also be very useful in exams when you are drawing on different types of memory and recalling knowledge from a wide range of sources. The subject material will evolve as you progress through medical school – being flexible and open-minded will ensure that you are ready to evolve with it.

# 1.3 **Cope with information overload**

Medicine, to all intents and purposes, is an infinite and ever-expanding subject. Even if you knew **absolutely everything** there was to know about medicine right now, every time you went to sleep there would be thousands of new studies published, rendering your knowledge out of date by the time you woke up.

Researchers have actually quantified this phenomenon by looking at how many different journals you would need to read to keep up to date with the major new research published in a single specialty in a single year.[4] They found that in neurology alone, for example, you would need to read a staggering 896 (yes, that's eight hundred and ninety six) different journals. To stay up to date in psychiatry, you'd have to read 545 journals; in oncology, 503 and in cardiology 374 (pity the poor GP who is somehow expected to know all of these different specialties!) Another group has tracked the steady growth of medical information since the 1940s, finding that well over a million articles are now published every year and growing fast (**Figure 1.1**).[5] Feel that brain exploding yet? I don't blame you (**Figure 1.2**).

I tell you this to illustrate that you are simply **never** going to be able to know everything there is to know about medicine. It is literally impossible and you should not try! Accepting and making your peace with this fact will help you cope with information overload – an unpleasant but unavoidable sensation which begins on day one of medical school and continues until you retire, die or both. Expect it and be ready for it.

Information overload feels particularly acute in the early years, when the sheer volume of material you are expected to learn seems utterly, crushingly overwhelming. Do not let this stress you out: by recognising it early, you can learn to cope with it. And remember that doctors are humans too, and they have also had to face this problem: no matter how knowledgeable and intimidating that neurosurgeon seems now, she also began medical school as a total ignoramus whose head span the first time she was told the corticospinal tracts decussate in the pyramids of the medulla (the what does what in the **what** now?). Now she's drilling through skulls and clipping aneurysms whilst absent-mindedly pondering what she's going to have for lunch. One day, you might be doing this too.

---

4 *BMJ*, 2012;344:e3223
5 Gillam, M. *et al.* 'The healthcare singularity and the age of semantic medicine' (pp. 57–64) in Hey, T., Tansley, S. and Tolle, K (eds) (2009) *The Fourth Paradigm: data-intensive scientific discovery.*

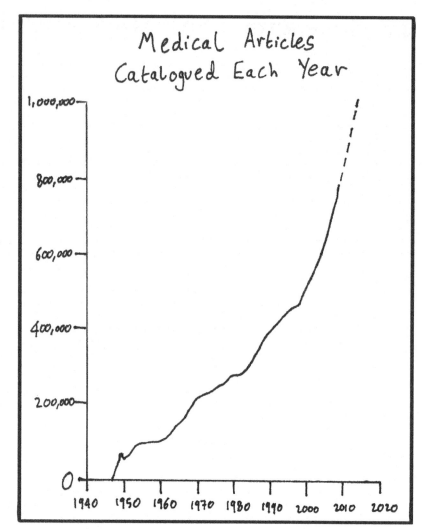

**Figure 1.1: The number of medical articles published each year has been rising sharply since 2000 and is thought to have recently passed the one million mark** – graph redrawn from data in Hey *et al.* (2009).[5] No human being on earth can handle this much information, so you will need to develop coping strategies and be selective about what you do and don't attempt to learn.

# 1.4  Use chunks and yield

With information overload in mind, it becomes super-important to get into the habit of **chunking**: breaking subjects down into digestible nuggets which you can work through piece by piece. This makes vast topics feel far less daunting, and allows you to steadily accumulate knowledge piece by piece, until one day you wake up and realise you have enough of it to become an FY1 doctor.

Let's say, for example, you decide to devote a study morning in first year to the intimidating topic of haematology. It's an entire specialty – where to even begin? You skim and decide that the two topics you want to cover are the structure and function of red blood cells and a brief overview of

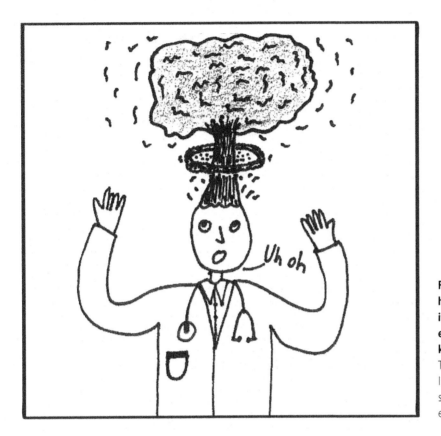

**Figure 1.2: What will happen to your brain if you attempt to learn everything there is to know about medicine.** Trust me, you will feel like this a lot at medical school, particularly in the early years.

common types of anaemia. These are nice, manageable chunks – you can devote two hours to each and still finish in time for lunch. Everything else can wait until tomorrow. Even if you don't finish, that's two topics you know **better** than you did when you woke up that morning. And that is an excellent start! This is a much smarter approach than just blindly ploughing into a haematology textbook, trying to cover something from every chapter and inevitably getting overwhelmed and demoralised.

Just as important as chunking is the concept of **high versus low yield**. This is the simple yet crucial idea that some topics are more worthy of your time and brainpower than others. After all, there's no point chunking if you can't prioritise the chunks! High-yield topics are those that come up often and carry lots of marks in exams; low-yield is the reverse. In haematology, for example, the topics mentioned in the previous paragraph are high yield for medical students; Waldenström's macroglobulinaemia, Fanconi's anaemia and the role of JAK2 mutations in polycythaemia vera are low-yield. And if you have absolutely no idea what I'm talking about, well, that's exactly my point.

> **Two critical concepts for surviving the onslaught of information coming your way in the next 4–6 years:**
> * **Chunking:** breaking large topics down into smaller, more digestible nuggets which you can process one by one.
> * **Yield:** recognising which topics come up most often in exams, carry the most marks and are therefore most important to cover.

To be clear: I'm not saying low-yield topics aren't interesting or important. Rare diseases, for example, are often extremely interesting and they are certainly important to patients who suffer from them and specialists who treat them. Just keep in mind that they are far less likely to come up in your exams than the more common stuff, and therefore do not represent the most efficient use of your time as a medical student. You can't cover everything, so you need to prioritise.

Chunking and yield are absolutely core skills for surviving medical school and ensuring you don't get drowned in information. We will revisit these concepts throughout this book.

# 1.5 Master time management

Studying for up to six years for a degree can do weird things to your sense of time, particularly at the beginning when it feels like an almost infinite expanse stretching ahead of you. One of the greatest challenges of medical school is to conquer this feeling of infiniteness by taking control of your time, breaking it into manageable pieces and treating it like a valuable resource. Respect it, don't waste it.

> Succeeding at medical school isn't about how much free time you have to study, it's all about how you use it. I am living proof of this fact! Having studied medicine whilst having two young kids, a long commute and a ton of other commitments, I managed to get distinctions and merits throughout, with far less time to study than most other students.

Time management comes very easily to some people and much less easily to others. If it is something you struggle with, I would advise getting some help and advice early on from your university or friends. Doing so will help you in so many ways: you can beat boredom, study more effectively, do better in exams and OSCEs and, most importantly of all, carve out enough personal time to keep yourself healthy, sane and in touch with friends and family. Improving your time management skills is also excellent preparation for being a junior doctor, when you will have a never-ending list of tasks and responsibilities which need prioritising and completing.

> Studying in short bursts can be extremely effective. Don't wait until you have several free hours in which to study, or you will miss countless opportunities to make the most of smaller, shorter slots.

**TOP TIP**

I will offer lots of time management strategies as we go along, but first and foremost I want to debunk the pervasive idea that you need hours of free time in which to study. This is nonsense: in fact, you can learn something in one minute, you can learn lots of things in 15 minutes, and you can learn **loads** of things in one hour. It just takes a little forward planning and careful selection of which resources are best to use. Flashcards, for example, lend themselves particularly well to short bursts of studying for up to 15 minutes at a time before you start to glaze over. With half an hour, you could re-read notes you have written previously or do some MCQs. An hour would allow you to skim a short book chapter, compile a table or sketch out some anatomy drawings. So don't wait until you have a whole morning or afternoon going spare – just grab whatever time you have available and make the most of it.

# 1.6 **Spiralise yourself**

Time to introduce another important concept: spiral learning. This is a classic bit of jargon that got bandied about loads at my medical school before anyone properly explained what it meant. Essentially the concept is simple: you learn a subject in brief then put it aside, then return to it later to add more detail then put it aside again, then return to it again in more detail, and so on (as opposed to trying to learn a subject in great detail first time around). It's supposed to resemble climbing a spiral staircase, although I think of it more like painting a wall: you do one layer, then leave it to dry before you add another. You can add as many layers as you like, but the point is to do the foundation coat properly and leave it alone for a while before attempting to put any more on top. If you try to paint all the layers at once the whole thing will end up as a soggy, sorry mess.

Once someone actually explained this concept to me, I found it very useful throughout medical school – both as a study technique and a coping strategy. Take renal medicine: one of the most daunting and confusing topics for medical students (and a lot of doctors!). You can easily get overwhelmed when your first lecturer, in a well-meaning attempt to provide a broad overview of the whole specialty, whizzes from the anatomy of the nephron to the pathophysiology of acute kidney injury, before delivering the knockout blow: glomerular diseases (if you don't know what these are yet, just take my word that they are fiendishly complicated and almost universally loathed by medical students). It all seems so abstract and complicated, particularly as you can't actually *see* any of it with the naked eye.

So approach it in layers, starting at the bottom with the absolute basics. In first year, your base coat could be simply to learn what the kidneys look like, where they are, what they do, and roughly how they do it. Your next coat, in second year, could be to gain a very broad understanding of what happens when the kidneys malfunction, both acutely and chronically. In third year you could layer on more detail about acute kidney injury, chronic kidney disease and the interpretation of renal function tests (three extremely high-yield topics). In fourth year, you could add a splash of end-stage renal disease, dialysis and transplants. And in final year the pièce de résistance: glomerular diseases, polycystic kidney disease and the effects of medications on the kidneys. It all feels much more manageable when broken down like this, as you are putting far less pressure on yourself to know it all straight away. Be happy to learn the basics properly and build up slowly from there!

**KEY POINT**

> Spiral learning means covering the basics of a subject first, then returning to it later to add a little more detail. This is a great way to learn and doubles up as a coping strategy to avoid information overload.

# 1.7  Go broad

Maybe you want to be a maxillofacial surgeon. You already studied dentistry, and know with cast-iron certainty that you wish to devote your career to developing a new system for staging oral cancers. If so, that's amazing and I wish you absolutely every luck with that endeavour! But first, you've got to get through medical school, and unfortunately your interest is pretty niche at this stage. In fact there is potential for it to be a hindrance – distracting you from higher-yield topics and dragging down your marks.

Because like it or loathe it, the best strategy for succeeding at medical school is to go broad – as broad as possible – rather than getting bogged down in the details of one particular subject.

**Faced with a choice, it's better to cover three topics in 6/10 detail than one topic 10/10. Most medical schools aim to produce graduates with wide general knowledge, so this approach will help get you through exams and OSCEs and provide the best preparation for life as a junior doctor.**

We all have inherent biases towards particular topics – but you need to be disciplined about them to ensure you cover everything else too. Recognise your interests and disinterests, and don't let them steer you off course. Make the most of broad placements like GP, acute medicine, general surgery, accident and emergency, intensive care and anaesthetics, and try to see patients with a huge range of conditions. You might indeed become a world leader in maxfax one day, but first you need to learn about diabetes, polycystic ovarian syndrome and diarrhoea, no matter how boring you find it!

Be aware of which topics you naturally gravitate towards and do not let them distract you from other important subjects. The best strategy for doing well at medical school is to have a broad general knowledge, rather than fixating on certain areas.

**TOP TIP**

# 1.8 Never be afraid to get stuff wrong

Perfectionist tendencies are a common trait among medical students and I was certainly no different at the start. We dislike getting things wrong, being shown up by someone else's knowledge, or being made to feel stupid or ignorant. By the end of my first clinical year, I could have reeled off a long and detailed list of times I had answered consultants' questions wrongly and felt a sting of wounded pride.

But I slowly came to realise what now seems obvious – that this sting, although unpleasant, had caused these incidents to lodge firmly in my memory. Hours and hours of medical school are spent trying to make information stick in our brains, often unsuccessfully, yet here I had stumbled upon a method for instantly imprinting an episode into my neural circuitry. It's the holy grail for students! All I had to do was attach the *correct* answer to the memory (this is usually easy, as the episode also involves the consultant telling you the correct answer with a sigh of disappointment) and hey presto, I'd actually learned something!

Even now I can effortlessly recall the definition of a hernia. Why? Because I got it wrong and had an exasperated GI surgeon grill me on it until I could reel it off word perfect. I remember that abdominal pain, vomiting and dizziness can be a presentation of Addison's disease, because I completely fluffed this in an OSCE station. And I know that deteriorating cognition in an elderly person with recurrent falls can point to a subdural haematoma, because a neurosurgery registrar told me so after I bumbled my way through presenting the case to him with no clue what the correct diagnosis was (Me: I think the patient has dementia. Registrar: Okay, so why is he on a neurosurgery ward? Me: He has, like, **really bad** dementia?).

**Never be demoralised by getting stuff wrong,
because it can be an amazing way to learn.**

In fact, these episodes are often **easier** to remember than the times you got something right. This seems counterintuitive, but it was absolutely true for me. So next time a consultant gives you a hard time for not knowing something, just take a deep breath, remember the unpleasant sensation of being made to feel silly, then go away and learn it. You'll know the answer the next time – and hopefully for years to come.

# 1.9  You *think* you know, but how do you *know* you know?

Studying medicine will play some really strange tricks on your brain. There's the one where you convince yourself you're harbouring whichever nasty disease you're learning about that week (aka medical student syndrome), the one where you forget your own name just as you begin introducing yourself in an OSCE station, and the one where your hands turn into giant clumsy hams the minute you're asked to do a procedure with someone watching you.

But the most common – and potentially damaging to your studies – is the 'Oh yeah, I totally know that' phenomenon. It goes like this: you spend a load of time studying something, to the point where you feel completely comfortable and confident with it. Then you're asked to recall the knowledge under pressure and suddenly your mind goes completely and utterly blank: is it duodenal or gastric ulcers that improve after eating? Was the cut-off 11 or 12 for diagnosing diabetes? And what the hell are those clotting factors blocked by warfarin again? I've witnessed this terrible affliction strike me and others more times than I can even begin to count. "Err… err… damn, I spent all of last night studying that and now I can't remember a bloody thing!" (*Figure 1.3*).

The way to alleviate this is to not just passively study a topic, but to keep **actively testing yourself** on it. I found it helpful to regularly ask myself: "okay, you *think* you know that topic, but how do you **know** you know it?" Then I would imagine myself bring grilled by a consultant, and challenge myself to clearly demonstrate the knowledge to prove that I really knew it.

There are many, many techniques for testing yourself, but one great way is to take a blank piece of paper and write down the key facts entirely from memory, without looking at your notes. Then get your notes out and mark your effort in red pen – throw the sheet in the bin and do it again and again until you can get everything right. This technique is especially good for covering anatomy (try drawing the biliary tree or the coronary circulation from memory) and physiological pathways such as the clotting cascade or bilirubin metabolism.

Another great option is to mentally rehearse explaining the knowledge to someone who knows nothing about it. Imagine you're in a busy noisy pub, competing for your friend's attention, and you have just 2 minutes to tell them everything about sepsis before they get bored and wander off to play pool instead. This technique should also help you be concise and convey the most pertinent points first, as well as testing the knowledge itself.

**Figure 1.3: No matter how well you can recall information in the comfort of your own home, it's an entirely different ballgame to do so under pressure.** You might *think* you know something, but it's of little use if you can't recall it when you need it the most.

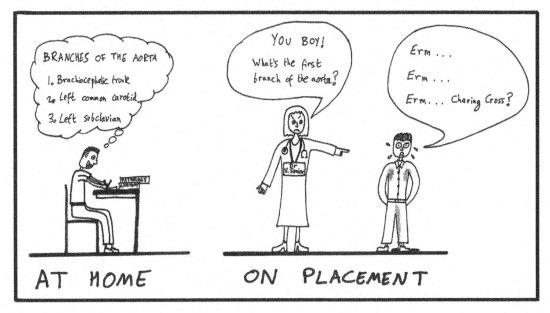

We will look at more techniques for self-testing as we progress through this book. I can't promise to **completely** banish 'Oh yeah, I totally know that' phenomenon, but I guarantee that this will at least make it a **whole lot** easier to recall knowledge under pressure.

**KEY POINT**

It's extremely common for information to completely vacate your brain when you are under pressure. Anticipate and prepare for this by testing yourself as you go along to ensure you really know the material properly.

# 1.10 **Learn to love language**

I love the English language. I suggest you learn to love it too. Because words are indescribably important in medicine, and there is simply no getting away from them, no matter how hard you try.

This might sound obvious, yet there is a tendency among many medical students to overlook the importance of language and communication in becoming a doctor. These people emphasise the development of practical skills and the accumulation of pure knowledge, and see communication skills as simply a by-product, or a means to those ends. I would argue that you will perform much better at medical school if you make improving your communication skills an end in itself.

**TOP TIP**

Pay close attention to the meaning of all the new medical words you learn and work hard on improving your communication skills. You'll do much better in OSCEs and on placements as a result.

Take OSCEs, for example – a subject we will return to many times throughout this book. You might think they are all about showing off your practical skills and examination techniques, about palpating, percussing and auscultating under the pressure of an examiner's watchful gaze. It might surprise you to learn, therefore, that 12 out of 15 OSCE stations in my medical school finals were in fact centred on communications rather than examinations or practical skills. Nine of these were history-taking stations and three were pure communication skills, such as breaking bad news or explaining a medication to a patient.

Imagine two robots taking this OSCE. One is a headless body built by the world's best mechanical engineers to possess superhuman skills – it can smell early-stage cancers, hear murmurs from the end of the corridor and insert a cannula with one hand while measuring blood pressure with the other. The other is simply a talking head, built by the brightest minds in linguistics, artificial intelligence and diagnostic reasoning. The disembodied head would charm its way through 12 stations, pass the exam and make national headlines by graduating as a doctor. The headless body would dazzle in three stations, crash and burn in the rest and find itself consigned to the historical scrapbook.

Of course as a medical student you want to be both the head **and** the body, but my point is that it would be a foolhardy strategy to neglect one skill set in favour of the other. And it's not just in OSCEs where words matter: you'll find anatomy easier if you pay attention to the names of things, blood-taking easier if you chat to the patient to put them at ease, and surgery more enjoyable if you take a history from the patient before the procedure. Ultimately, you will be a better doctor if you can work on improving your linguistic and communication skills throughout medical school and beyond.

# 1.11  Be a team player

Medicine is a team sport: patients do better when their healthcare professionals all pull in the same direction, and worse when individuals strike out on their own. The same goes for being a student: it helps enormously to set your stall out early as someone who cooperates with their peers. You will quickly find that you reap what you sow: share great resources you have discovered, and others will share right back at you. Study in groups, and you will benefit from new ideas and fresh perspectives on a topic. Help out those who are struggling, and someone will help you out when you're in need.

Sadly, you will almost certainly encounter students who do the opposite: they are overly competitive, they hoard knowledge, they put others down. You need to take a deep breath and rise above these antics, safe in the knowledge that yours is the better long-term strategy for success at medical school and beyond.

# 1.12  Recognise patterns

Forget Archimedes and his bath – for me, the real Eureka moment came in my second year of medical school when a lecturer told us that the vast majority of medical practice is essentially just pattern recognition. This extremely simple idea had not previously occurred to me, and I think it's something every student should consider from day one. It's absolutely critical.

Pattern recognition explains why doctors seem so impressive the first time you observe them at work. How on earth does that GP know the patient has osteoarthritis within 30 seconds of beginning the history? Because they've seen osteoarthritis **thousands** of times before, and they recognise that this is how it usually presents. How on earth can that paediatric cardiologist so easily distinguish a VSD from a PDA, when you can barely even remember what the letters stand for? Because they've seen more congenital heart defects than you've had hot dinners, and **this is what they sound like**.

Understanding this concept serves two purposes. First, it's a great coping strategy when you are finding things overwhelming: of course you can't instantly recognise that murmur because **you've never heard it before**, so go easy on yourself! Secondly, it provides great impetus for your studying, by reminding you that you need to build up your own bank of experience from which you can start to recognise patterns. So the best way to get good at detecting murmurs is … drum roll … to go and listen to as many murmurs as you can! Want to be able to confidently diagnose osteoarthritis? Speak to patients with osteoarthritis! You'll never recognise these patterns if you spend all day with your head buried in textbooks.

**KEY POINT**

Pattern recognition is absolutely essential to the practice of medicine. I cannot emphasise this point enough! Develop yours by getting hands-on at every opportunity, looking at hundreds of results and scans, doing as many examinations and taking as many histories as you possibly can.

Quite quickly, once you are aware of it, you will feel your pattern recognition begin to grow and develop. It's especially noticeable with physical examinations – if you've seen or heard something before, you will spot it much faster second time around, and even faster the third. It's immensely satisfying on clinical placements when, for the first time, you can say: "I actually know what this is because I saw it last week". It's even better when this happens in an OSCE. Pattern recognition is absolutely key for reading investigations such as ECGs and chest X-rays, and also comes into its own with written exam questions – by doing hundreds of them, you will start to instinctively recognise certain phrases and keywords which quickly give away the answer (**Figure 1.4**). And when that happens, your hard work will be really paying off.

# 1.13  Flip reverse it

As part of constantly testing your knowledge, you should always try to flip facts around and approach them from multiple different directions. **Box 1.1**

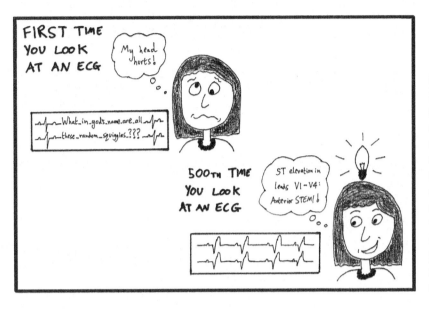

**Figure 1.4: Pattern recognition plays an absolutely crucial role in medicine and you will need to develop your skills through practice and experience.** ECGs are a great example of this: only by looking at hundreds of them can you hope to make any sense of all those weird squiggly lines.

shows an example, using the high-yield topic of the arterial territories involved in stroke:[6]

Use this technique whenever you are mentally rehearsing a topic. Don't be happy with just reciting knowledge to yourself in one particular way – make sure you approach the same piece of knowledge from multiple different angles. This ensures that you really do know the material properly and helps you avoid being caught off guard by sneakily worded questions.

**Box 1.1**

---

**Example of flip reversing a piece of knowledge**

Original order:
*Q: Which motor centres does the anterior cerebral artery predominantly supply?*
*A: Lower limbs*

Once you can answer that from memory, it's time to flip it around:
*Q: Which artery predominantly supplies the lower limb motor centres?*
*A: Anterior cerebral artery*

Got that? Flip it again:
*Q: A patient presents with acute-onset leg weakness. Which artery is most likely to have been affected?*
*A:  Anterior cerebral artery*

And so on...

---

6 *Medicine in a Minute*, p. 221.

# 1.14  Take a deep breath and count to ten...

Despite your best efforts and intentions, medical school won't always go to plan. Lecturers will fail to show up, clinics will be cancelled and tutors will go on holiday without anyone telling you. You'll get to the library nice and early to 'get in the zone' before an exam, only to discover workmen drilling directly above the silent study area. Books will get lost, tablets will crash, new clothes will get blood on them and coffee machines will break precisely when you need them most. You can deploy all of the techniques described in this book and more, yet there will still be occasions when you're not learning anything and feel like you're wasting your time.

**TOP TIP**   Medical school involves plenty of frustration and disappointment. Take a deep breath, count to ten and move on.

The best you can do is accept that some amount of frustration is inevitable, and learn to cope with it. If nothing else, this will prepare you well for working in the NHS! You might like to take a deep breath and count to ten, or tell yourself to BAM (breathe, accept, move on). However you do it, just make sure you develop some sort of coping mechanism for when things fall short of expectations or fail entirely. Because it simply isn't worth expending vast amounts of your energy getting worked up about it. You'll tire yourself out. Tomorrow is another day – reset yourself and be ready to go again.

# 1.15  When in doubt, DIY

So much of medical school is about getting things to 'stick' in your brain – to transform words and pictures into memories you can actually use when you need them. The best way – sometimes the only way – to master this is **to do things yourself** instead of relying on other people's work. You don't need to be an expert on human memory to appreciate that information just sticks better if you have invested your own time and effort into it.

A common example: you show up to a tutorial and your friend has made an amazing one-page summary of common causes of hearing loss. It has bright colours, perfect pictures and information so masterfully chunked that even your granny could understand it. Your friend is a team player, so kindly lets you photocopy it. What next?

Creating your own learning materials will help information to stick in your brain *far* better than just using stuff someone else made.

**TOP TIP**

Well, if you're anything like me, you could spend hours admiring that page and still fall squarely into the trap outlined in **Section 1.9**. Unless you have a true photographic memory (lucky you!), I would urge you instead to make your own version – taking the time to read, think about and understand each little bit. Reword any bits that don't make sense to you, cross-check against your own notes and make sure the facts are accurate. This might seem laborious but trust me: an hour spent doing something yourself is far better than an hour spent admiring something someone else made.

This principle applies to almost any information you study, be it online videos, anatomy textbooks or a lecturer's slides. Don't just stare at it hoping it will go into your brain, because it won't! You need to customise it, personalise it, create your own materials from it. You'll remember things so much better that way. And if you remember them better, you can recall them more easily when the time comes.

# 1.16  Figure out your med school flavour

I talked to a lot of people about their experiences of medical school while writing this book. And one of the things that struck me most was just **how much** variation there is in the style and content of medical degrees, particularly in the preclinical years.

Some universities – the more traditional ones, shall we say – place enormous emphasis on learning basic sciences such as anatomy, physiology and pathology. They will expect you to know every muscle, bone and nerve in the body, to learn complex biochemical pathways entirely off by heart and to know the detailed structure and function of bacteria, viruses and fungi. They might even expect you to have a detailed understanding of embryology: the science of how humans get formed right from the moment when sperm meets egg. It doesn't matter whether or not this information will help you when you graduate and become an FY1 doctor (most of it won't), but they'll expect you to know it anyway!

Different medical schools have very different priorities, agendas and teaching styles. It's helpful to figure out yours, so you can adapt yourself accordingly.

**KEY POINT**

Other universities have modernised and taken a more pragmatic approach by focusing their medical degrees on the things that newly qualified doctors need to know to get on with the job. These schools tend to emphasise clinical and communication skills and problem solving. They try to ensure all the science is rooted in understanding real patients: they won't expect you to recite obscure scientific facts and concepts just for the sake of it.

There are pros and cons to each approach, but there's little point debating these because at this stage you've presumably already accepted your place so you're stuck with whatever you've got! But I would encourage you to try to discover and think about the 'flavour' of your medical school, particularly in the early months, so that you know what to expect and can adapt your approach accordingly. If they strongly emphasise basic science, then brace yourself for a lot of rote learning and recitation of facts. If the emphasis is more clinical, then group study, role play and placements will come to the fore.

**TOP TIP** Make friends with students in the years above. They will give you great insights about what to expect and which subjects your medical school tends to emphasise in exams.

# 1.17 If you can, teach

One of the best, best, best tips I can give you for medical school is to take up any opportunities to teach students in years below you. This usually takes the form of helping run anatomy sessions in the dissection room, or being a clinical skills tutor (I did this). But there may be other options at your medical school, or even chances just to teach informally through societies or on clinical placements. Whatever the opportunities are, take them, because it's incredible revision and you will learn a huge amount.

Why is teaching so great? First, it gives you the opportunity to revisit and consolidate the knowledge in your head before explaining it. Then your knowledge gets reinforced and strengthened by repetition each time you run the same session. Finally, you get the benefit of seeing other people learn the topic for themselves, seeing what mistakes they make and why, which in turn further reinforces the knowledge in your head. It's a really efficient use of time and makes information stick in a way that few other methods can match. Teaching is also fun, sociable and a great way to meet students in different year groups. I really cannot recommend it highly enough!

# Chapter 2
# **Preclinical years**

## Contents:

# 2.1 What's it all about?

For most readers, coming straight from school, your first years of medical school are when you finally get to be a proper student. There will be people to meet, sports to play, drinks to down, societies to join and endless other temptations and distractions. This can be an incredibly exciting period in life, particularly if you are living away from home for the first time, and I strongly encourage you to explore new opportunities and enjoy yourself.

But I'm not here to tell you how to run your social life – you've got Instagram for that. I'm far more interested in the small matter of, you know, passing your medical degree and becoming a doctor. So at the same time, I must urge you to find the right balance between having a good time and learning stuff, so that alongside all the partying you are also setting yourself up properly for the clinical years and beyond (**Figure 2.1**).

The great news is that, at this stage, medicine feels new and exciting and studying can be a lot of fun. Every medical school does things differently but generally speaking, you will have between one and three years to focus on learning the 'basic sciences' (this is a stupid name as they are complex

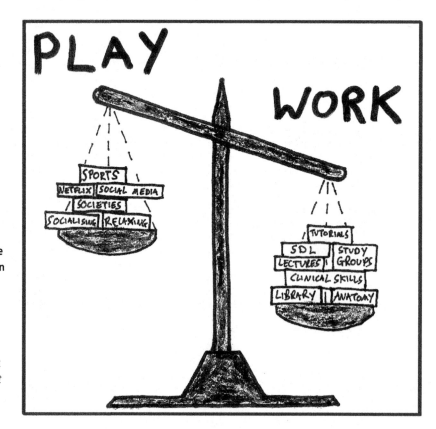

**Figure 2.1: Finding the right balance between work and play can be a challenge in the preclinical years.** You can load plenty of stuff onto the fun side – and indeed you *should* – but make sure the scales *just about* tip in the right direction.

subjects and there is absolutely nothing basic about them!). The big three are anatomy, physiology and pathology, plus there'll be varying amounts of biochemistry, pharmacology, embryology, molecular biology, histology, epidemiology and statistics thrown in for good measure. You'll almost certainly have some ethics, professionalism and law too, plus clinical and communication skills, depending on how early your medical school likes to introduce these.

So essentially, these years are about learning how the body works, why people get sick and what doctors can do about it. And the thing about the human body is – it's absolutely awesome. These are the years when you can indulge your fascination and delve deep into subjects: marvel at the intricate anatomy of the hand, puzzle over the pathophysiology of leukaemia or scratch your head discovering how neurons communicate with one another. You may not realise it yet but you have a lot more time to study in these years than you will at any other point of medical school, and probably a lot more passion too! So in this chapter we'll look at how you can maximise all that time and channel all that enthusiasm into studying effectively, while still making enough time and space for your personal life. I hope that by doing so, you can expand your knowledge at great speed while keeping yourself fresh and excited about medicine.

## 2.2  Why bother?

In many ways, you are now a student just like any other. And like other students, you may be hoping to scrape through with maximum fun and minimum effort – doing just enough to pass each year and ensure you make it over the finish line. After all, a doctor who graduates bottom of the class is still a doctor, right?

Well yes, but there are also some important differences that come with training to become a doctor. I mean, there's that whole sense of ethical and professional duty: the idea that you are entering a higher calling and that society will expect more of you than, say, a history of art graduate. Or the fact there is more riding on your academic performance than for most students: one day you will be treating real people, and they might actually suffer harm if you don't know your subject properly. No one's going to die if a geography graduate can't remember how oxbow lakes are formed.

These arguments are all well and good, but there's also a far more down-to-earth reason why as a medic you should aspire to getting good marks: it will have an absolutely **massive** impact on how and where you spend the years of your life following medical school. Once you graduate, you will

**Unlike other university degrees, your marks throughout medical school will influence where you live and work for at least two years after you graduate. Eek.**

**KEY POINT**

Don't rely on the SJT to drag up your score for application to the UK Foundation Programme. You have more control over your medical school performance, so try to do as well as possible in *all* your exams.

apply for your first two years of jobs through a national, centralised system called the UK Foundation Programme. It's a competitive process in which everyone is given a score out of 100, almost half of which is based on your academic performance ***throughout*** medical school (***Figure 2.2***), not just at finals (the other half comes from the Situational Judgement Test; we will discuss this and the Foundation Programme in more detail in ***Chapter 5***).

In other words: do well every year, ace the SJT and you can take your pick of jobs in the locations, hospitals and specialties that you desire. Coast through and you might find yourself miles from home working in lousy departments doing jobs you're not suited to. Of course there is potential to drag your marks up with a strong performance in the SJT but this is a stand-alone, one-off exam: there is unpredictability to your performance on the day, so you cannot ***rely*** on it. You have much more control over the academic component, so in my opinion the best strategy is to make your academic score as strong as possible by doing well throughout medical school (there's also the fact that high marks and distinctions can help you out later with applications to specialty training, as we'll see in ***Section 3.7***).

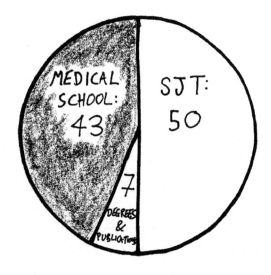

**Figure 2.2: Scoring system for entry to the UK Foundation Programme.**
Your medical school performance is worth 43 out of 100 points, then your 'educational achievements' (publications and other degrees) are worth another 7 points. Together these are known as the Educational Performance Measure (EPM), worth 50 points in total. The remaining 50 points come from the Situational Judgement Test (SJT), a one-off exam focusing on professionalism, ethics and law.

I'm not trying to scare you but I think most medical students genuinely don't realise this fact: they think that if they scrape through the early years they will still have the opportunity to lift their game later on, in time to get good jobs. But it doesn't always work like that because, in my med school at least, our results from each year carried the exact same weight as each other. And final year marks didn't even count towards the Foundation Programme! So there was just as much to be gained from bossing your first year as your fourth year, for example, and nothing to gain from prioritising final year over earlier years. For me, this was *the* major reason to get my ass into gear from year one.

Not all medical schools work like this though: some six-year degrees, for example, only count your performance in years 4 and 5 towards Foundation Programme applications. So if you feel strongly about where and how you will work after you graduate, make sure to check the website and course handbook for your medical school to find out how much weight they give to each academic year when calculating Foundation Programme scores. You may well discover that the start of first year is a good time to begin making an effort!

> Find out how your medical school calculates the scores for the academic performance part of the EPM. This will allow you to plan and prioritise your studies. If they give equal weight to each year, then it's a good idea to start taking things seriously from your very first set of exams. If first year doesn't count towards the EPM, then there is less pressure and you can ease yourself into it.

**TOP TIP**

## 2.3 What are you trying to achieve in the preclinical years?

Before you take the plunge and bury your head in the books, it is helpful to think about what you are trying to achieve during your preclinical years. Essentially you are trying to build up a huge amount of knowledge in a short space of time: to go from knowing virtually nothing about medicine to knowing enough about all of the different body systems and diseases that you are ready to enter your clinical years and be unleashed on an unsuspecting public.

I want you to think of this like an epic building project (*Figure 2.3*). Your GCSEs and A levels were the foundations, and now you have an empty plot of land on which to build an enormous, awesome skyscraper. Believe me, it's going to make the Empire State Building look like some amateur arts and crafts project by comparison. To pull this off, however, you can't just start throwing concrete around; you need to carefully consider the different components and how they fit together:

1. **Knowledge:** this forms the bricks of your skyscraper. The bricks are the main part of the structure – they give it shape, form and height. But bricks don't just stick together all by themselves...

2. **Techniques:** these form the cement that joins your bricks together. By using different techniques to study effectively, you ensure that the bricks hold fast and allow your skyscraper to rise up from the ground without collapsing.

3. **Resources:** these are the tools and equipment you use to apply the cement to the bricks. After all, what use are the world's finest bricks and cement if you've got no way to apply one to the other?

These three elements – knowledge, techniques and resources – are the absolutely critical core components you need to build your skyscraper and succeed at medical school. This is important to appreciate because in my experience, med students tend to fixate on knowledge without thinking as carefully about the other two. Whatever topic they are learning about, they dive straight into reading about it or watching a YouTube tutorial and just hope desperately that the information will stick in their brain. But this is generally ineffective, because the information will inevitably fade over time if it isn't properly reinforced. In other words, these students are eagerly stacking up the bricks of anatomy, physiology, biochemistry and so on, but without the right tools and cement the structure just slowly collapses, leaving them with a pile of bricks rather than a skyscraper. They are constantly having to go back over topics they already covered, which is frustrating and an inefficient use of time.

For these reasons, my focus in this chapter is not teaching you the knowledge part of medicine, because you have an army of lecturers, entire libraries of books and the infinite vastness of the internet to do that. Instead we will focus more on techniques and resources, which are every bit as important but don't get nearly as much airtime.

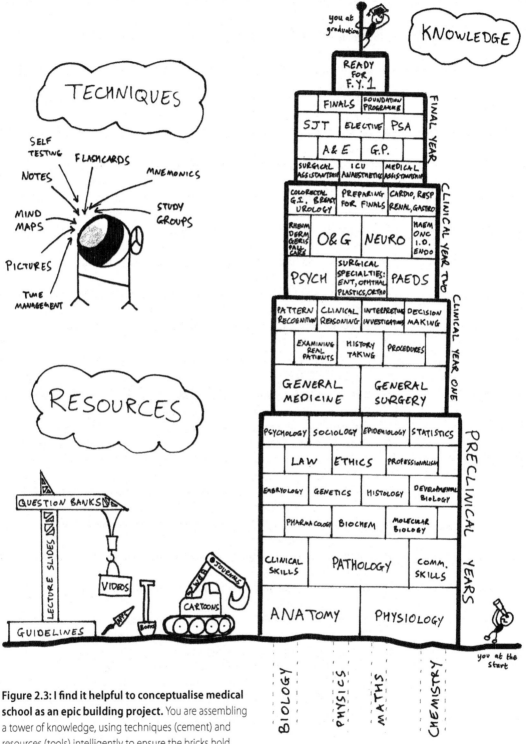

**Figure 2.3: I find it helpful to conceptualise medical school as an epic building project.** You are assembling a tower of knowledge, using techniques (cement) and resources (tools) intelligently to ensure the bricks hold fast without collapsing. You will need all three of these elements – knowledge, technique and resources – to support the other; none is much use in isolation.

**How to study effectively in the preclinical years** (see sections in brackets for more detail):

- Appreciate the concept of spiral learning and use it to build up your skyscraper of knowledge (*Sections 1.6* and *2.3*).
- Flip reverse your knowledge – always make sure you can approach information from multiple different angles (*Section 1.13*).
- Study *actively* – keep your brain engaged and make sure information is going in (*Section 2.6.3*).
- Test yourself again and again and again to make sure you actually *know* stuff instead of just *thinking* you know it (*Section 1.9*).
- Experiment with a wide range of techniques and resources, customise them and develop your own, then focus in on approaches that work well for you (*Sections 2.4* and *2.5*).
- Take control of your time and use it wisely (*Section 2.6.1*).
- Get into good habits: minimise distractions, take breaks and look after yourself (*Section 2.6.2*).
- Be organised and have a good filing system so you can find things you need. Hang onto great resources or notes you have written so you can come back to them in later years (*Section 2.6.2*).
- Take the 'fluff' seriously (*Section 2.6.4*).

**Box 2.1**

### Common pitfalls in the preclinical years

- Fixation on knowledge without considering the techniques and resources needed to acquire and retain it.
- Having a very narrow view of how to study and not experimenting with new methods.
- Not matching techniques and resources to the topic you are studying.
- Neglecting high-yield topics or over-focusing on low-yield topics.
- Poor time management and organisational skills.
- Obsession with the idea that you need several free hours to study, then failing to use shorter slots.
- When you do get a long free period to study, getting bored and falling asleep in the library.
- Getting stressed and overwhelmed (although this is very understandable!).
- Not looking after yourself properly, or burning out early.
- Thinking you know a subject better than you really do, because you haven't flip reversed it or tested yourself properly on it.
- Not realising your marks will impact Foundation Programme applications.
- Doing everything alone instead of studying in groups, helping out your peers and being a team player.
- Studying passively by letting information wash over you without making sure it is actually sticking in your brain.
- Neglecting subjects perceived as 'soft', such as communication skills, ethics, professionalism and law.

# 2.4  Study techniques

So you know you need to study, but exactly **how** do you go about it? Clearly there is no magic answer to this question: everyone is different, and you will need to work out for yourself through trial and error what your best approach to studying is. But what I would strongly suggest at this early stage, with a bit of time on your hands, is that you experiment as much as possible. Don't just assume that what worked for you at school will continue to work for you forever! Try new ways of doing things, no matter how weird they seem at first, and ask other people for their ideas and inspiration about ways to study. I certainly surprised myself – I knew from my previous degree that I was a massive notes writer, for example, but it was only through other people's influence and a bit of experimentation that I came to love flashcards and study groups in medical school. Keep an open mind, and you might surprise yourself too.

Here, therefore, are the main techniques which I used to study at medical school and would recommend you give a try. Of course this list is not exhaustive – there are infinite different ways to study – but try to use these as a starting point, in combination with the resources listed in **Section 2.5**. Challenge yourself to try all of these in your first term and come up with even more of your own. There really is no limit: I've seen people invent games, songs and even dances to help them remember stuff. If it works for you then go for it!

## 2.4.1  Notes

Whether you write by hand or type, use swathes of bright colours or pure monochrome – there is no escaping the fact that you will need to generate your own notes in order to get through the preclinical years. This is probably the technique that comes most naturally to students: you will instinctively know how to do it and will probably just crack on with it from day one. But don't simply stick to whatever you did before: take the opportunity to try different things. Maybe you always typed your notes – why not try writing by hand on paper for a change? See **Table 2.1** for some pros and cons to each approach. Why not use loads of colours instead of black and white? Try embedding pictures into your notes instead of keeping them separate?

However you go about writing them, there are five things you should always do to maximise the value of your notes:

1. **Look at them again:** let's say you wrote ten pages of notes during a lecture on the menstrual cycle. Don't just file them away, never to be seen again! Take them out the next day and re-read them while the topic is still fresh in your mind. This helps the content to sink in and ensures you didn't waste your time.

2. **Customise them:** that paragraph you wrote about the role of different hormones throughout the cycle – wouldn't that look better as a graph? If so, draw it and stick it in! And if that bit you wrote about the luteal phase feels incomplete … get your pen out and add to it! Don't treat your notes as sacred and untouchable – you can keep adding and tinkering to your heart's content.

3. **Rewrite them:** if those ten pages have become 20, covered in scribbles and scraggly Post-it notes, perhaps it's time to throw them out and start again. This is a great chance to freshen them up with a little editing – keep in the best bits, scrap the rubbish bits, add in extra pictures you found online and hey presto, you've got yourself a brand new set of Menstrual Cycle Notes 2.0. This process of editing and rewriting also really helps the information stick in your brain.

4. **Summarise them:** challenge yourself to turn any set of notes into a mind map or one-page summary of 'everything you need to know about the menstrual cycle'. You'll be amazed by how much you can condense the information. Then you can rehearse and reinforce the knowledge by glancing at the key headings in your summary and mentally filling in the rest.

5. **Test yourself on them:** once you've got your notes looking beautiful, try to test yourself on them as often as you can. Cover up a section and try to mentally recall the information; write a short essay summarising all the key points then mark it against your notes; or attempt some MCQs (multiple choice questions) from a textbook. However you do it, testing yourself will help transfer the information from notes to brain and ensure your time was well spent.

**TOP TIP**

Five ways to get maximum value from any notes you write:
1. Look at them again while they're fresh in your mind
2. Customise them
3. Rewrite them
4. Condense and summarise them
5. Test yourself on them

Table 2.1: The pros and cons of electronic vs. paper notes

|  | Pros | Cons |
|---|---|---|
| **Electronic** | • Quicker to write<br><br>• Edit as you go along<br><br>• Easily copy and paste chunks of text, insert pictures and links, compile information from multiple different sources<br><br>• Anyone can read them<br><br>• Easy to access, swap and share<br><br>• Switch formats, e.g. turn your notes into electronic flashcards or MCQs | • Information just doesn't seem to 'stick' as well in your brain<br><br>• By copying and pasting things, you sometimes forget to actually read and think about them<br><br>• Need to carry your laptop around<br><br>• Risks of technical failure, Wi-Fi outage, flat battery, etc.<br><br>• More potential distractions from notifications and messages<br><br>• Higher electricity bills |
| **Paper** | • Information seems to go into your brain better than when you type it<br><br>• Material in your own handwriting feels more familiar<br><br>• Can't take shortcuts by copying and pasting – you need to actually think about what you're writing<br><br>• Hand-drawing pictures can be strangely therapeutic | • Slower to write<br><br>• Folders take up a ton of space<br><br>• Not always easy to access<br><br>• Need a good filing system so you can find things when you want them<br><br>• Handwriting needs to be legible<br><br>• Environmental impact of paper consumption |

## 2.4.2 Drawings

Next time you're in a tutorial, sneak a cheeky glance at other people's notes. Chances are, you'll find there's a closet Michelangelo in your midst. It blew my mind when I saw how amazing some students' drawings were: lifelike renditions of the human body in a stunning array of colours. My drawings, on the other hand, were a bit rubbish: 8/10 for effort, 3/10 for achievement. However, this doesn't seem to have held me back – in fact my loose and unscientific observations of my peers suggest that there is no correlation whatsoever between drawing ability and performance as a medical student.

So if you're like me, or worse, **_do not be put off_**.

**Drawing is an absolutely fantastic technique for learning medicine, no matter how lousy the actual pictures are. You learn from the process, not from the end product.**

Indeed there are loads of topics that can't really be learnt any other way. Take hormone loops from endocrinology as a classic example (*Figure 2.4*): these would take hundreds of words to write out, and even then you probably wouldn't understand them as clearly as in pictures. And this type of basic schematic is delightfully simple to draw, no matter how bad at art you are, so there really is no excuse not to try! Your drawings don't need to be complex: you can always simplify things down to basic lines and shapes, which can be easily knocked together with a biro or in Microsoft Word or PowerPoint. Alternatively, you can trace around pictures from anatomy

**Figure 2.4: Thyroid function pathways.** Hand-drawn, basic schematics like this are nice and easy to remember and will save you a lot of time compared to writing everything out in words.

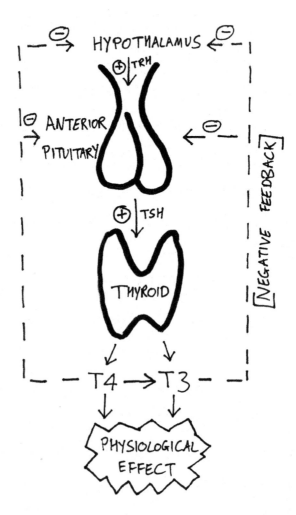

books then annotate and colour them in yourself (I did this a lot – it makes your notes look much more impressive than they really are).

The other great thing about drawing is that it can feel rather relaxing and therapeutic, particularly when you are frazzled from other study techniques. Drawing feels like doing something different, so it provides some welcome variety and can really help to break up long study sessions and keep you feeling fresh. There is even a whole range of anatomy colouring books for people who really enjoy this sort of thing – I would urge you to give it a try!

**Subjects that lend themselves to drawing as a study technique**           **Box 2.2**

- Anatomy: either detailed drawings or tracings, or simplifications down to schematic form.
- Physiology: biochemical pathways involving multiple organs and chemical messengers can almost always be simplified into a nice schematic, e.g. hormone feedback loops, bilirubin metabolism or the clotting cascade.
- Histology: no matter how fiddly it looks down a microscope, you can almost always turn it into a nice simple picture.
- Summarising guidelines and algorithms for diagnosis or treatment.

## 2.4.3 Tables

As we have just seen, you'll quickly find there are many topics in medicine that simply don't work well as long passages of text. If you are finding a topic dry, and your notes are getting too long, ask yourself: could this work better as a table? Chances are you'll find the information much easier to digest that way. I drew absolutely loads of tables and boxes in my notes, particularly when I wanted to summarise and condense a lot of information into a smaller space or group things into categories (see **Table 2.2**). Once you've drawn a table you can easily use it for self-testing: just redraw the empty frame and challenge yourself to fill in the details without looking at the original (**Table 2.3**). Tables are also great for when you need to compare and contrast different points, such as in **Table 2.4.**

**Table 2.2: Assessment of asthma attack severity: an example of condensing a lot of knowledge into a small, more manageable table[1]**

| Severity | Clinical features |
|---|---|
| Moderate | • Increasing symptoms<br>• PEF >50% best or predicted<br>• No features of acute severe asthma |
| Acute severe | Any one of:<br>• PEF 33–50% best or predicted<br>• Respiratory rate ≥25/min<br>• Heart rate ≥110/min<br>• Inability to complete sentences in one breath |
| Life-threatening | Severe asthma with any one of:<br>• PEF <33% best or predicted<br>• $SpO_2$ <92%<br>• $PaO_2$ <8kPa<br>• Normal $PaCO_2$ (4.6–6.0 kPa)<br>• Silent chest<br>• Cyanosis<br>• Poor respiratory effort<br>• Arrhythmia<br>• Exhaustion, altered conscious level<br>• Hypotension |
| Near-fatal | Raised $PaCO_2$ and/or requiring mechanical ventilation with raised inflation pressures |

1 British Guideline on the Management of Asthma: www.sign.ac.uk/sign-153-british-guideline-on-the-management-of-asthma.html

**Table 2.3: Once you've compiled a table, you can test yourself by filling in a blank version without looking at the original**

| Severity | Clinical features |
|---|---|
| Moderate | 1.<br><br>2.<br><br>3. |
| Acute severe | Any one of:<br><br>1.<br><br>2.<br><br>3.<br><br>4. |
| Life-threatening | Severe asthma with any one of:<br><br>1.<br><br>2.<br><br>3.<br><br>4.<br><br>5.<br><br>6.<br><br>7.<br><br>8.<br><br>9.<br><br>10. |
| Near-fatal | 1. |

## 2.4.4 Mind maps

Mind maps, aka concept maps or spider diagrams, are another great technique which is rightly popular among medical students. They are a superb way to make a subject more visually appealing, easier to remember and for summarising and condensing a whole topic into a single page, particularly when the topic has lots of overlapping or interconnecting ideas. See *Figure 2.5* for an example from my first-year notes. You don't have to hand-draw them, although personally I liked doing so: there are loads of apps, websites and books devoted to mind mapping. Look in your app store, Google it or ask your friends which ones they use, then have a play around and find whichever works best for you.

**Table 2.4: Ulcerative colitis vs. Crohn's disease – an example of using a table to compare and contrast two similar conditions.** This is a particularly high-yield topic which comes up *a lot* in exams, and they will expect you to know exactly which of the two conditions is being described. A table is a useful way to frame the side-by-side comparison and get the differences straight in your head.[2]

| | Ulcerative colitis | Crohn's disease |
|---|---|---|
| **In a nutshell** | Most common type of inflammatory bowel disease. Unknown aetiology. Relapsing-remitting course. | Second most common type of inflammatory bowel disease, also of unknown aetiology. |
| **Typically affects** | Men and women of any age but peaks at 15–30 and 55–65 | Slightly more common in women. Any age but peaks at 15–20 and 60–80 |
| **Anatomy** | Affects the rectum and spreads proximally | Affects any part of the GI tract, particularly the terminal ileum |
| **Histology** | Wide, shallow ulcers. Inflammation is continuous and affects mucosa only. | Deep, fissuring ulcers with granulomas and stricture formation. Inflammation is not continuous (skip lesion and cobblestone patterns) and affects all layers of GI tract. |
| **Clinical features** | Bloody diarrhoea, abdominal pain, rectal bleeding | Diarrhoea (not always bloody), abdominal pain, rectal bleeding, weight loss, ulcers and fistulae |
| **Extra-intestinal manifestations** | Common to both: finger clubbing, erythema nodosum, pyoderma gangrenosum, arthritis, anterior uveitis and episcleritis | |
| | Primary sclerosing cholangitis and cholangiocarcinoma | Mouth ulcers, gallstones, nutritional deficiencies |
| **Effect of smoking** | Improves symptoms | Worsens symptoms |

Another great way to use mind maps is for testing yourself on topics you have already covered. Start by copying out the mind map leaving just the headings in place, then challenge yourself to fill in the bubbles without looking back at the original map or your notes (**Figure 2.6**). If you can do that successfully, your next step is to work your way up to drawing the entire mind map purely from memory. Once you can do that – you're flying.

## 2.4.5 Flashcards

I have a confession to make: I *love* flashcards. If there was an 'I ♥ flashcards' T-shirt, I would wear it every day for the rest of my life. I quite possibly love flashcards more than my own children. Heck, I would have named my daughter Flashcard if my wife would have allowed it. I realise this makes me a deeply tragic person but I don't care because without

---

2 Sources: my notes and flashcards (original sources unknown) and *Medicine in a Minute*

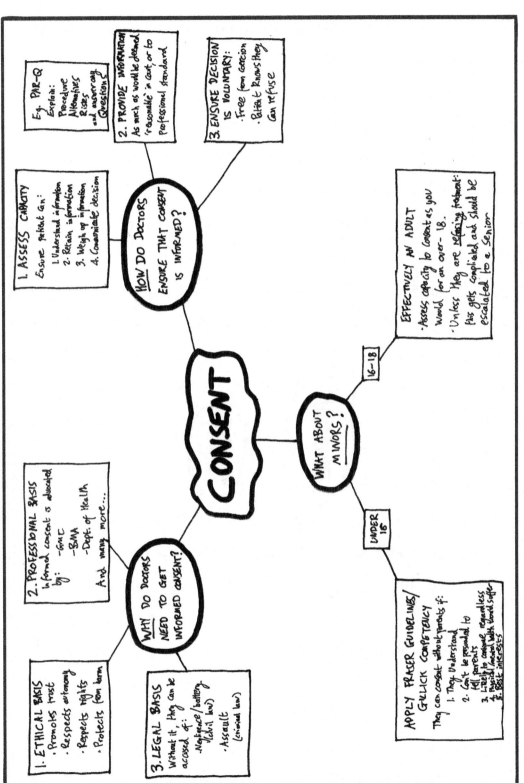

**Figure 2.5: Example of a mind map for studying the important topic of consent.**

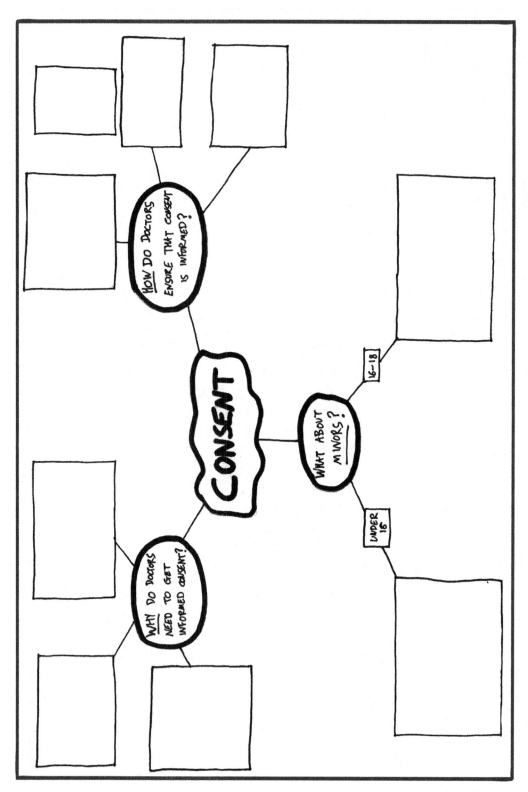

Figure 2.6: Use blank mind maps like this as a way to test yourself on the subject by filling it in without looking at the original.

flashcards I'd probably still be in medical school, endlessly repeating first year and crying into my LOBs. **So there**. I feel much better now that's off my chest.

Why are flashcards so amazing? Because they tick **SO** many boxes as an effective study technique:

- They are versatile and can be used for almost any topic, from the anatomy of the lumbar spine to the sections of the Mental Health Act.

- They can be used for very short bursts of studying, even just a few minutes at a time.

- They are a very **active** form of studying, particularly if you build your own cards, and they work well alongside any other study technique.

- They are a fantastic method for testing yourself, and encourage lots of quickfire repetition and reinforcement of knowledge.

- They combine words and pictures to test different aspects of your memory.

- Their small size requires concise, snappy summaries without unnecessary waffle.

- They are portable and fit in your pocket, so can be used anywhere at any time (I have studied flashcards in bed, on trains and planes, even at the Emirates Stadium while waiting for an Arsenal game to start).

- They are endlessly versatile: you can make infinite different combinations and keep chopping and changing to your heart's desire.

- They let you flip reverse your knowledge by approaching it from different angles.

Flashcards come in three different forms: pre-made ones such as Netter's Anatomy Flash Cards (see **Section 2.5.3**), handmade ones where you draw/ write them yourself onto little cards, and electronic. Pre-made flashcards are especially brilliant for studying anatomy as the pictures are often too complex to draw for yourself, and you can test yourself by trying to name all the different structures without looking at the answers. If making your own, whatever the topic, the main point is to ensure that there are questions of some form on one side of the card and answers on the other so that you can test yourself properly while keeping the answers hidden. If you put all the information onto a single side of the card then you have essentially just produced a miniature summary of your notes – this is fine if that's what you intended, but for me the key element of flashcards is the ability to do quickfire self-testing and to rapidly flick between the questions and answers.

Electronic flashcards require a little more explanation as you may not be familiar with this technique. I used a clever app called Flashcards (there are absolutely tons on the market; see **Section 2.5.4**) on my phone and tablet, which harnesses a learning technique called 'spaced repetition' to help you memorise stuff effectively. **Figure 2.7** shows you how it works. This approach forces you to keep confronting your weak areas by repeatedly serving you the questions you find most difficult, while sparing you the easy ones. Google 'spaced repetition' if you want to know more of the theory!

**KEY POINT**

Flashcards are one of my favourite methods for self-testing and reinforcing knowledge. They come in three forms:
1. Pre-made – great for studying anatomy and physiology
2. Handmade – great for testing yourself on your notes
3. Electronic – great for anything and everything.

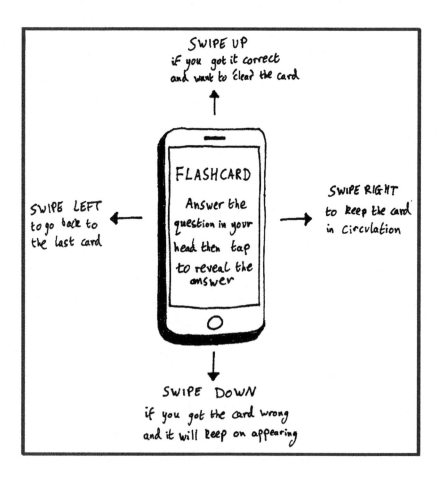

**Figure 2.7: How to operate electronic flashcards using spaced repetition.** Same skills as Tinder, substantially lower payoff.

That's how it works, but first you need to build the actual flashcards. I did this in Excel spreadsheets: it's super-easy, you just create one column for the question and another for the answer (**Table 2.5**). Once you import it into the app you can add pictures and even sounds to each flashcard, so that you are essentially building a completely personalised, interactive medical quiz. Make one 'deck' of cards for cardiology, another for respiratory, and so on, depending on whatever you are studying that week. The decks can be as large or small as you like, fiendishly complex or super-basic, according to your tastes. Add in pictures from absolutely anywhere: illustrations from books, things you drew yourself or screenshots from videos of websites (**Figure 2.8**). Be creative! This process does take a bit of time but it's so worthwhile as you're creating an extremely valuable learning resource which you can dip in and out of as you please. And they will last you for years: I used mine all through medical school, customising the decks each year by adding in a bunch of new questions, dropping the ones that had become too easy, and keeping the ones I still found difficult.

The beauty of electronic flashcards is the constant repetition and reinforcement which builds up your pattern recognition: do a short session every day and you will find the information **really** starts to stick. This approach is especially brilliant in the run-up to exams and OSCEs when you want the information to pop straight to the front of your mind with minimal thinking and retrieval time.

**Table 2.5: Example of some of my electronic flashcards from the early years of medical school, as written in a very simple two-column spreadsheet.** Upload this to your flashcards app and you're ready to roll.

| Question | Answer |
|---|---|
| What is the formula for calculating cardiac output? | Cardiac output = heart rate × stroke volume |
| Define a true vs. false aneurysm | True: a localised, permanent, abnormal dilatation of a blood vessel by more than 1.5 times its normal diameter. Lined by endothelium.<br><br>False: a haematoma which is continuous with vessel lumen. The endothelium is broken and does not line the inside of the aneurysm. |
| Give four causes of a petechial rash and some specific examples of each | 1. Infection: septic emboli, invasion of capillary walls or immune complex deposition: bacterial (esp. meningocci, streptococci, *H. influenzae*) or viral (e.g. measles)<br><br>2. Haematological: impaired haemostasis: thrombocytopenia or platelet dysfunction<br><br>3. Vascular: vasculitis, scurvy, drugs<br><br>4. Mechanical: capillary injury: local pressure, strangulation, coughing or vomiting |

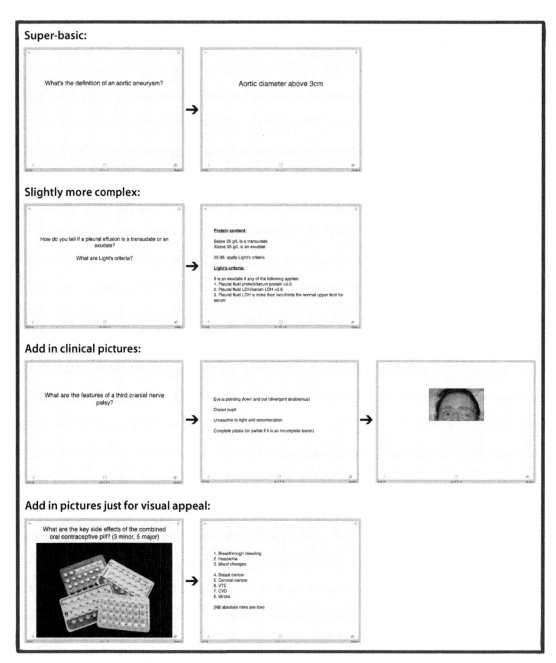

**Figure 2.8: Example screenshots of electronic flashcards as they appear in use with the 'Flashcards' app.** These are just a handful of the hundreds I made during medical school. You can customise them to your heart's content, adding pictures and even sounds such as heart murmurs.

## 2.4.6 Structured frameworks

You've probably never heard of Dr Deac Pimp but he is a very old friend of mine who helped me a lot through medical school. He will help you too, so please allow me to introduce him.

Dr Deac Pimp is a structured framework for learning about any disease (*Figure 2.9*). It's a mnemonic which stands for: **D**efinition, **R**isk factors, **D**ifferential diagnoses, **E**pidemiology, **A**etiology, **C**linical presentation, **P**athophysiology, **I**nvestigations, **M**anagement and **P**rognosis. Okay, the abbreviation is lame (don't blame me – I didn't invent it), but stick with it because Dr P is a truly excellent method for enhancing your learning in the early stages of medical school. Any time you encounter a disease you are unfamiliar with, be it COPD, HIV or melanoma, you can work your way through these ten essential points and you will find they give you a brilliant overview of the topic. In fact, they essentially cover everything you need to know about a disease in order to pass medical school finals!

The advantage of this approach is that it provides a clear order for you to work through a subject piece by piece, in a systematic way. It makes new topics seem less daunting and takes a lot of the hassle out of knowing

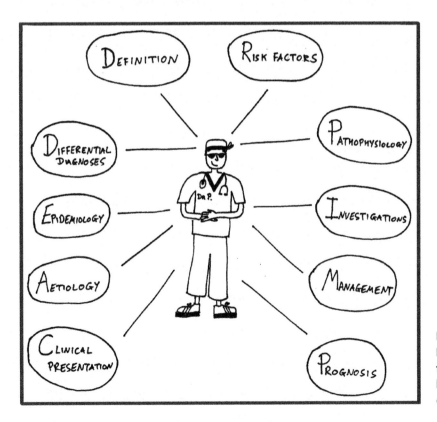

**Figure 2.9: Dr Deac Pimp is a structured framework for learning about any disease.**

where to start your research, because you know **exactly** where to start: with a definition, then risk factors, and so on. You can just get straight on with researching it, safe in the knowledge you'll cover all the main points. And once you've completed a Dr Deac Pimp on a topic, it's easy to revise from as it is already chunked so you can easily test yourself on one bite-sized section at a time. It's also easy to convert the information into tables, mind maps and flashcards, or to divide the sections up between members of a study group to present each one in turn.

In no way do I claim to have invented Dr Deac Pimp (kudos to whoever did), but I certainly used him a **lot** in the preclinical years. I'm sure there are plenty of equally excellent alternatives in circulation – whichever you choose, just be systematic and you will find it makes large topics seem much more accessible and easier to digest. We will look at lots of other structured frameworks throughout this book which are helpful for organising your thoughts, including surgical sieves and formulae for approaching clinical examinations.

**KEY POINT**

Structured approaches such as Dr Deac Pimp are useful for studying preclinical topics because they:
- Ensure you are thorough, systematic and don't miss important bits
- Make big subjects feel more accessible
- Help you know exactly where to start when researching a new topic
- Keep the information tidy in your brain and help it stick better
- Facilitate revision and self-testing
- Are easy to convert into mind maps, tables and flashcards.

### 2.4.7 Mnemonics

As well as giving you a structure to study from, the letters of Dr Deac Pimp are also a type of mnemonic device. This is defined by the Oxford English Dictionary as something "designed to aid the memory" – basically any approach you use to help you remember stuff better. You've probably already used mnemonics to get through your A levels, and you will encounter many, many more throughout med school. Some medical mnemonics have been around for donkey's years, used and loved by thousands of students; others your mate just made up on the spot and are simply never going to catch on, no matter how enthusiastic they are about it. I am not going to attempt a comprehensive list here – there are entire books devoted to medical mnemonics – but have suggested a few classic examples in **Box 2.3**. Some have been sanitised due to crude language!

**Some classic medical school mnemonics**

Box 2.3

Causes of pancreatitis: **I GET SMASHED**
**I**diopathic, **G**allstones, **E**thanol, **T**rauma, **S**teroids, **M**umps, **A**utoimmune, **S**corpion sting, **H**igh triglycerides, **E**RCP, **D**rugs

Functions of the 12 cranial nerves: **Some Say Money Matters, But My Brother Says Big Brains Matter More**
**S**ensory, **S**ensory, **M**otor, **M**otor, **B**oth, **M**otor, **B**oth, **S**ensory, **B**oth, **B**oth, **M**otor, **M**otor

Branches of the external carotid artery: **Some Anatomists Like Freaking Out Poor Medical Students**
**S**uperior thyroid, **A**scending pharyngeal, **L**ingual, **F**acial, **O**ccipital, **P**osterior auricular, **M**axillary, **S**uperficial temporal

Carpal bones of the hand: **Some Lovers Try Positions That They Can't Handle**
**S**caphoid, **L**unate, **T**riquetrum, **P**isiform, **T**rapezium, **T**rapezoid, **C**apitate, **H**amate

I'm a huge fan of using mnemonics at med school simply because the volume of information you are expected to remember is so huge, that anything you can do to make it easier has got to be worthwhile! They also really help you out when you are trying to recall information under pressure: you'll typically find the mnemonic jumps into your head much quicker than the individual bits of information. Even if you can't remember what **all** the letters stand for, you should at least be able to make a start. You can also build mnemonics into your notes, flashcards and mind maps to help you remember chunks of information.

Mnemonics are a very personal thing: you will love some and hate others. Be on the lookout for them from day one, invent your own if possible and make an effort to write down and remember any good ones so that you can start building up your own mental collection. And of course there are many different types of mnemonic: people come up with dances, chants, songs and even weird finger movements to help them remember stuff. Whatever works for you!

Mnemonics are potentially brilliant but you do need to be a bit discerning: if you are really struggling to remember what all the letters stand for, then by definition it's a rubbish mnemonic and you shouldn't waste brain space on it!

TOP TIP

## 2.4.8 Study groups

To my mind, study groups are an absolute **must** for medical students. I'm talking about informal groups where you get together with a few friends on a regular basis and study together. There is absolutely no way I would have got the marks I did were it not for being part of some fantastic study groups during the early years of medical school. I had three separate groups on the go: one for covering academic content, one for clinical skills and one for pharmacology. This is a substantial time commitment but trust me, it is absolutely worth every second! Here's why I love them so much:

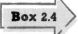
**Box 2.4**

**The advantages of study groups**

- Sociable and fun way to learn.
- Chance to swap resources, techniques and ideas.
- Test and reinforce subjects you have already covered by yourself.
- Calibrate your knowledge against others'.
- Provide structure and regular deadlines of topics to revise.
- Nice variety from self-directed learning.
- Helps keep you sane (-ish).
- Good excuse for some serious snackage.

Setting up a study group is easy, but be sure to pick people you get on well with and with whom you can study effectively. They don't have to be your best friends or housemates: in fact it might even be a good idea to reach out of your immediate circle in order to bring some variety and fresh perspectives to the table. Remember that you're not organising a social club or a night out here: the goal is to enhance your studying, so the priority is to find people who will support that aim. People who are flaky and unreliable, lazy or expect others to do all the work for them are not good partners for a study group, no matter how much you love them or how funny they are. Try to limit the numbers so that everyone can remain engaged and get lots of chances to contribute: between three and six people is probably ideal.

Once you've assembled your crew, make sure everyone knows what it's all about and how often you are going to meet up. Aim for once a week, timetable permitting, for a couple of hours somewhere with a whiteboard, pens, internet access and plenty of snacks to keep you going (it ain't no study group if there ain't no hummus). Choose topics in advance so that everyone has a chance to go over them in good time.

**Try to meet up weekly with your study
group and go over material you were taught
a few weeks previously, to ensure it remains
in your mind rather than fading away.**

There are infinite different ways to run study groups, but here's how we did it:

- Each week, follow the curriculum from around four weeks earlier: i.e. study group in the first week of October covers everything you were taught in the first week of September; in the second week of October you cover the second week of September, and so on. This is a nice time lag so that the material is still present in your brain but is just starting to fade out (your goal is to stop that from happening!). What's more, this comprehensive structure is important as it forces you to cover **everything**, instead of just randomly picking whatever subjects you enjoyed and ignoring the ones you didn't.

- Have a clear list of objectives for each session, preferably based on the official LOBs (learning objectives; see **Section 2.4.9**). Our university provided LOBs on a weekly basis, which made this easy, but you can devise your own list if required.

- Everyone needs to prep by looking over all the LOBs by themselves. Obviously people will be stronger on some topics than others, but in theory **everyone** should know a little about **every LOB**.

- When you meet, randomly divide up the LOBs between each person. Then go through the list taking it in turns to present/explain your LOB to the whole group for a few minutes, using plenty of whiteboard drawings.

- Have your notes handy but try **not** to look at them while presenting to the group. Be polite and respectful and don't interrupt other people while they are presenting!

- Have a few minutes of discussion after each presentation to share ideas, resolve points of difference and swap any good resources or techniques you found for that topic.

- Make sure you listen carefully to other people's presentations and learn from them. Spot gaps in your own knowledge and keep track of topics you will need to brush up on before exams. If someone had a great way of explaining something you hadn't previously understood, make a special effort to remember it so that you can recall it in exams.

### 2.4.9  Use LOBs to your advantage

My medical school was **very** hot on learning objectives, known as LOBs for short. These are essentially a way to break the curriculum down into bite-sized chunks of everything we needed to know. Although well intentioned, the trouble was the list of things we needed to know was so absolutely brain-bogglingly massive that the bite-sized chunks swiftly piled up into a festering food mountain so large that to even think about it would induce cyclical vomiting syndrome. Long lists of LOBs were dished out on a weekly basis, giving the sense that you were being constantly stalked by a malevolent shadow version of your mum nagging you to do your homework. No surprise that LOBs were not exactly popular among medical students.

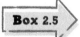
**Box 2.5**

**Examples of LOBs (learning objectives) from my preclinical years, selected at random from a list of hundreds**

- Describe the structure and movement of the joints of the forearm, wrist and hand.
- Identify the cranial nerves and the functions they serve.
- Outline the milestones of normal development in early childhood and methods for their assessment.
- Explain the value of randomised clinical trials in informing the management and prevention of diabetes.
- Describe the metabolism of bilirubin.
- Define angina and myocardial infarction.

However your med school decides to dress it up, the bottom line is that somewhere there is an extremely large, pre-determined list of all the topics you need to learn during your preclinical years. If this is drip-fed to you week by week, like it was for me, you will almost certainly find it annoying, but do consider that it is better than the alternative: I can only imagine how utterly terrifying it would be to receive an entire year's LOBs in one go. Either way, it is worth trying to suppress your fear and disgust to try to harness LOBs as a way to support your learning. Here are some of the ways you can use them to your advantage:

- Avoid wasting time on topics that aren't in your LOBs. If it ain't in there, they can't examine you on it!

- Identify high- and low-yield topics according to how much weight they are given in the LOBs list and how much they overlap with lecture and tutorial content

- Take a bird's eye view of the entire curriculum to ensure you're not getting too bogged down into individual topics

- Cross off LOBs as you go, to keep track of what you have learnt so far and where there are still gaps in your knowledge

- Plan self-directed study sessions more effectively by matching LOBs to particular resources or techniques

- Convert LOBs into flashcards (**Section 2.4.5**) or study group agendas (**Section 2.4.8**)

- Use LOBs when devising revision timetables to ensure you don't miss any topics (**Section 2.9.1**)

- If all else fails, you can always take your LOBs list down the end of the garden and ceremoniously set fire to it. It'll make you feel better for a short while, at least.

## 2.4.10  Test yourself again, again and again

Sometimes in life, you've got to love, nurture and be kind to yourself. Other times, you gotta look straight in that mirror and be a big old meanie bully who won't take any nonsense. Med school involves being both good cop and bad cop – but when it comes to testing yourself, you will need to be the latter.

Why? Because it is far too easy to convince yourself that you know a subject, particularly when you have spent several hours studying it. "Of course I know the structure of a nephron – duuuuh – there's that bit with the glomerulothingy and then the descending loop of whatsit and then the salt comes out and the water goes in and then weeeeeeeeeeeeeeeeeeeeeeeeee! Right?" No, mirror face. Not. Good. Enough.

The way around this is to **test yourself as you go along**, instead of waiting to get found out in your exams. Whenever you study, build in some time at the end for self-testing using the techniques listed below. It's normal to discover that you didn't know the topic as well as you thought you did – don't panic, just be aware of this and make sure you revisit it later and test yourself again. Repetition is the key: by testing yourself over and over and over, you will soon find that the information sticks. If you just look at it once and move on, it simply **will not**. So be hard on yourself and test, test and test again!

Box 2.6

**Testing techniques: how to assess your knowledge after a study session**

- Draw pictures, tables and mind maps entirely from memory, then mark yourself against the original. Throw your attempt away and repeat again and again until you can do it correctly from memory.
- Cover up your notes, run through the content in your head, then look at your notes again to see how much of it you actually knew.
- Explain/teach the topic to a friend without looking at your notes. Encourage them to ask you lots of questions, then be sure to look up the ones you couldn't answer later.
- If your friends aren't around, imagine how you would explain the topic to a random person you just met in a busy, noisy pub.
- Attempt some MCQs from a book or online question bank, or write your own (*Section 2.4.11*).
- Build some flashcards: keep repeating them until your performance improves.
- Look over the LOBs for that subject and ask yourself honestly whether you have achieved them.

## 2.4.11 Make your own MCQs and quizzes

When testing themselves, most students will instinctively turn to pre-existing questions such as in textbooks or an online question bank. This is all well and good; however, there is another great but largely under-used technique which is to **write your own questions instead**. I find this really reinforces your knowledge of a subject by making you distil it down to a series of key points and rearrange it into a new form. It's also a helpful exercise to come up with reasonable-sounding wrong answers as well as correct ones, as you can start to imagine the sort of traps that examiners might lay for you.

You can write questions just for yourself (you'll need to set them aside for a while so that you forget the answers before attempting them), or do it through a study group where you write questions for each other. Some students also write questions for online question banks, earning a little extra cash in the process. Another variation of this is to put together interactive online quizzes using software such as Mentimeter. Your audience logs in using their smartphones and completes your quiz live in real time, competing against each other. You can do this any time you have to give a presentation such as at student grand round, or you can do it informally in study groups. It's fun and engaging – your audience will love it – but crucially you will benefit loads too from the process of writing the questions and answers. Give it a try: you'll find it really helps the information to stick.

Try writing your own MCQs or an interactive quiz whenever you are studying a particular topic. This is a superb way to test your knowledge and create a resource which you can come back to as exams approach.

**TOP TIP**

## 2.4.12 Calibrate your knowledge

In **Section 2.4.8** I mentioned that study groups provide an opportunity to calibrate your knowledge against other people's. This concept is well worth understanding properly, so let's expand on it as a study technique in its own right.

As we discussed in **Chapter 1**, two of the biggest problems in the early years of medical school are dealing with information overload and learning how to identify and prioritise high-yield subjects. Calibration is one way of doing this: essentially you crowd-source the problem by finding out how much everyone else knows about a topic, then use that information to guide your own studies.

Immunology is a good example. We had a very long and complex series of lectures in first year about how the immune system functions, right down to the molecular structure of the human leucocyte antigen (HLA) system and major histocompatibility complex (MHC) proteins. A lot of this stuff made my head hurt: it all felt very technical, scientific and far removed from actual human beings. I had no idea how relevant it was and how much detail I needed to go into for my studies. This is a very common feeling in the preclinical years!

What you need to do is try to gauge the crowd: how much do your friends know about HLA and MHC? Is everyone else's head hurting or just yours? In all their study time, has anyone come across a practice question where this knowledge was **actually** required? This is another reason why study groups and small tutorials are so great: discussing a LOB together gives you an idea of how worthwhile everyone else considers it to be. If they've all put loads of work into it and know far more than you, then you should probably brush up on it. On the other hand, if you've gone into far more detail than anyone else, then perhaps you overdid it!

Calibrating your knowledge means using other students to figure out which subjects are important, high-yield and worthy of your time. If everyone seems to be taking a subject very seriously, it's probably important; if they're not, it probably isn't.

**KEY POINT**

Of course this strategy risks giving you a bum steer, leading you to neglect a topic which then features heavily in your exams. But more often than not, the wisdom of the crowd will prove to be correct, helping you to focus more effectively on high-yield topics. In this case, as it turned out, I did not need to know the intricacies of HLA or the MHC, nor the complement pathway or intracellular signalling in phagocytes for that matter. A fairly basic knowledge of T and B cells, neutrophils, antibodies and hypersensitivity reactions was perfectly sufficient for my preclinical exams!

### 2.4.13 Summary

In this section, we have looked at some study techniques to help you survive the preclinical years. These form the cement that holds your bricks of knowledge together. The key points are:

- Use a wide variety of different techniques to study including, but not limited to: notes, drawings, tables, mind maps, flashcards and LOBs.
- Try new things – don't just rely on what worked for you at school.
- Study with other people, take an interest in their ideas and approaches and calibrate your knowledge against theirs.
- Use structured frameworks and mnemonics to help you remember information.
- Write your own MCQs and quizzes.
- Always test and appraise your knowledge as you go along.

## 2.5  Study resources

As we discussed in **Section 2.1**, the preclinical years are primarily about building up your knowledge of the structure and function of the human body, in health and in disease. Your choice of resources will need to reflect this goal, focusing primarily on those big three subjects of anatomy, physiology and pathology.

Nowadays, thanks to the internet and smartphones, there is a near-infinite amount of information available to you at the tap of a finger. That is both a blessing and a curse: you have more choice and a wider diversity of information than ever before, but also a greater risk of misinformation from poor-quality sources. There is also huge potential to get overwhelmed by the sheer volume of material available, and suffer an acute exacerbation of information overload.

Perhaps the best strategy to cope with this is to allow yourself a period of experimentation at the beginning of medical school: try out loads of different resources, be open-minded and see what works for you. Then at some point you should start to narrow down and settle on your tried and trusted resources, so that you know exactly where to go to find the information you need. If you don't narrow down in this way, you risk being forever stuck in a kind of limbo where you can't learn the material effectively because you haven't found the right tools to do so. Ideally you should gradually reach a stage where you can dive straight into your 'go-to' books, websites and apps to tackle whichever topic you are learning that week, without wasting much time looking for the right resources.

With this in mind, let's look at a handful of the resources available to you. This is not – and could never be – an exhaustive list, but is intended just as a starting point from which you should cast your net far and wide! Your university should also have loads of suggestions to get you started.

> Experiment with using loads of different learning resources at the beginning of your preclinical years. Once you figure out your favourites, start to narrow down so that you know exactly where to look for particular types of information.

**TOP TIP**

## 2.5.1 Lecture slides

There is a good case to be made that these are **the most** important resource available to you at medical school. Not because they are necessarily the best quality or contain the most information, but because they are written by the people who compile your course and write your exam questions. By their very nature, they **have to** contain the information you need in order to pass the year, it's just a case of finding it. Any time you are struggling with information overload, you can look back at the lecture slides and use them to help you focus your studies: if the lecturer seemed fixated on a particular aspect of the topic – you should probably fixate on it too!

Now, there are some students who will tell you that lecture slides are **all** you need to get through medical school. Some will even go so far as to advise you not to bother attending lectures – just to work off the slides in your own time. Personally I disagree: I think there is enormous value in using a wide variety of resources to broaden your mind and keep your studies fresh and interesting. I mean, let's be honest, looking at PowerPoint gets boring pretty quickly! I also believe you will learn a lot more by looking at the slides **and** attending the lectures, not to mention the fact that poor attendance can get you into trouble. But I certainly agree that lecture slides are extremely important, and they should probably be your default starting point for any new topic you are studying. I'd suggest using them as a guide to figure out what you need to know about a topic, extracting the best bits, then turning to other resources to fill in the rest.

**Box 2.7**

> **Why are lecture slides so important?**
>
> - They're written by the same people who write your exams and OSCEs: look out for clues as to what's likely to come up.
> - The key information is almost always in there *somewhere*.
> - Can help you establish yield, i.e. figure out which topics to devote the most time and effort to.
> - Often contain great pictures and figures which you can put into your own notes and flashcards.
> - Use them to get the most out of lectures (**Section 2.6.5**).

## 2.5.2 Textbooks

See **Table 2.6** for some suggested textbooks for anatomy, physiology and pathology. These all have their own personalities and strengths and I am not specifically recommending any one over another: it is all a matter of personal taste as to which you use, so check them out for yourself. Do bear in mind the 'flavour' of your medical school (**Section 1.16**): for example, I used **Clinically Orientated Anatomy** because St George's is a very clinically focused medical school and exam questions were rumoured to be drawn from it! However, this book may not work as well for other med schools.

Anatomy books come in two different forms: textbooks and atlases (essentially just the pictures in larger form with less text). Textbooks are ideal for writing notes; atlases are great for drawing or tracing your own pictures. There is also a whole range of anatomy colouring books you might want to check out. Pharmacology is a topic we will look at in **Chapter 3**, but skip ahead for suggestions if you need to get stuck into it earlier. You may find *Rang & Dale's Pharmacology* useful at this stage: it is classically considered the leading textbook for pharmacology, but it is very large and has more of a scientific than clinical flavour so will be better suited to some medical schools than others.

Another option is to break topics down by medical specialty or body system. Each specialty has its own classics, too many to list here, but there are some great series which are worth checking out during the preclinical years, listed in **Box 2.8**. These tend to be smaller, more portable and easier to dip into than the classic anatomy, physiology and pathology textbooks.

A final word on textbooks: do not rush into buying particular ones just because your medical school tells you to, as you can waste a lot of cash on books which just sit on your shelf gathering dust.

> **Study resources are a very personal thing so you need to find out which textbooks you really like, enjoy and _actually use_ before investing money on them, particularly the massive and very expensive tomes which you will simply never manage to read from cover to cover.**

What's more, your med school's reading list may be out of date as there are new books being published all the time, including fresh and innovative texts to challenge the more 'classic', old-school titles. I'd suggest you spend a few weeks at the start exploring the library and trying loads of different books, then only buy ones you find yourself using regularly. I relied mostly on library loans and only bought around five textbooks throughout medical school, plus inheriting a few from friends and family and picking some up for free when signing up for various things such as medical indemnity cover. And you might very well discover you don't use textbooks to study at all – that's absolutely fine, so don't waste your money on them!

**Suggested series of textbooks which have multiple different editions**

 Box 2.8

- _Illustrated Colour Texts_
- _The ABC of ..._
- _... At a Glance_
- _Lecture Notes_
- _The Unofficial Guide to ..._
- _Essential ..._
- _The Oxford Handbooks_
- _Master Medicine_
- _Crash Course_

**Table 2.6: Suggested textbooks for the major preclinical subjects**

| Subject | Books |
|---------|-------|
| Anatomy | • *Netter's Clinical Anatomy*<br>• *Gray's Anatomy*<br>• *Grant's Atlas of Anatomy*<br>• *Clinically Orientated Anatomy*<br>• Any anatomy colouring books |
| Physiology | • *Guyton and Hall Textbook of Medical Physiology*<br>• *Tortora's Principles of Anatomy & Physiology* |
| Pathology | • *Robbins and Cotran Pathologic Basis of Disease*<br>• *Underwood's Pathology*<br>• *Pathoma*<br>• *Muir's Textbook of Pathology* |

## 2.5.3 Pre-made flashcards

The leader in pre-made, hard-copy flashcards is Netter's, which has separate series covering anatomy, physiology and neuroscience. However, there are loads of others for all sorts of subjects, including Brenner's Pharmacology Flashcards, Rang & Dale's Pharmacology Flashcards, the Oxford Handbooks Clinical Tutor Study Cards, and the Lange series, to name but a few. Again, don't rush to buy these until you are sure this approach is for you. But personally I bought the Netter's Anatomy and Neuroscience flashcards early on and got phenomenally good use out of them, right the way through medical school.

## 2.5.4 Electronic flashcards

I built mine in Excel then ran them through a fairly basic app called Flashcards. However, there are absolutely tons of apps and websites out there. Some allow you to build your own from scratch; others have pre-made electronic decks which you can download and run.

**Flashcard apps and websites**

- Flashcards
- Flashcards+
- Quizlet
- AnkiApp
- Brainscape
- www.almostadoctor.co.uk/flashcards
- www.cram.com/medical
- Medical FlashNotes
- Daily Anatomy Flashcards
- Instant Anatomy Flash Cards
- Lange series

## 2.5.5 Online video tutorials

There are some absolutely brilliant tutorials available for free online: you could probably find videos to cover your entire curriculum if you looked hard enough. My personal favourites were Khan Academy, Handwritten Tutorials, Dr Najeeb and Armando Hasudungan. Make sure you give these a try: they can be long but some of their explanations are fantastic, particularly for simplifying difficult concepts. Just make sure you study actively (**Section 2.6.3**) while watching videos: make notes and sketches, repeat information back to yourself, keep pausing and going back over things you didn't understand, and go through any summary material at the end. Don't just hit play, zone out and kid yourself that it counts as studying!

Check out these YouTube channels and websites for some superb tutorials in the preclinical years:
- Khan Academy
- Handwritten Tutorials
- Dr Najeeb
- Armando Hasudungan

## 2.5.6 DIY MCQs and quizzes

It's easy to write your own MCQs and quizzes using standard software such as Microsoft Word or PowerPoint, and involve your friends the old-fashioned way. But if you want to be more sophisticated and get them taking part through their smartphones, there are lots of cool programs such as Mentimeter, Typeform, Kahoot and MyQuiz. These generally allow you to make a basic quiz for free but will charge you for more sophisticated features, so ask whether your university has an institutional subscription which students can use.

## 2.5.7  Apps

See *Table 2.7* for the essential apps which you will use throughout medical school, as well as the flashcard apps we already mentioned. Beyond these, there are hundreds if not thousands of other medical apps – and growing fast – so be sure to keep checking what's new and exciting. If you can think of it, there is almost certainly an app for it! For the preclinical years, I was also a big fan of apps like Essential Anatomy which let you explore and play around with the human body in 3D – perfect for when you are struggling to make sense of a structure from your notes and pictures. There are also tons of apps for mind mapping, if it's your thing.

**Table 2.7: Essential apps for surviving medical school**

| | |
|---|---|
| • The *BNF*<br>• Microguide<br>• BMJ Best Practice<br>• UpToDate<br>• Geeky Medics | These really come into their own during the clinical years; however, they are still useful at this early stage and it is definitely worth getting to know your way around them as early as possible. Your medical school may subscribe to only one of BMJ Best Practice and UpToDate, so just go with whichever you can access for free. |

## 2.5.8 Question banks

Online question banks are going to be a mainstay of your studying over the next 4–6 years and we will discuss later how you can best use them to your advantage. The main players are PassMedicine, Pastest and OnExamination – each has its own look and feel, and various different features, so be sure to try them all out before settling on your favourite. You don't need to do anything fancy for now: just tell them your stage of medical school and they should be able to provide questions which are suitable and relevant to your learning. These are a fantastic way to test your knowledge once you have studied a topic.

My only caveat is that I would urge you to pace yourself: if you're anything like me, you will use online question banks more and more as you progress through medical school, and there is a risk you will make yourself sick of them if you peak too early! So it may be sensible to use them sparingly at this stage to keep your powder dry for later.

For other sources of questions, look up your favourite textbooks as they will often have companion websites packed full of quizzes and other helpful resources. Your medical school should also provide sample questions and/or mock exams to help you get a flavour for their specific style and wording of questions.

---

**Sources of practice exam questions**

- PassMedicine
- PasTest
- OnExamination
- Dedicated MCQ book series such as *Get Ahead, Oxford Assess and Progress* and *Single Best Answers in Medicine/Surgery*
- Most textbooks have a question section at the back or on an accompanying website
- Practice papers from your medical school
- Write your own

 Box 2.10

---

## 2.5.9 Websites

In the preclinical years you are often approaching a topic with absolutely zero knowledge, so will instinctively do what any sensible person does nowadays and just Google it. Wikipedia will of course figure prominently in the results and – shhhh, don't go telling your esteemed professors – you'll realise that the quality of medical information on there is actually surprisingly good and appropriate for your stage of learning. The NHS website is also a great starting point for any topic, and the professionals section of Patient.info is excellent (they have started charging for some content though). Try Medscape if you are going into depth on one particular disease, as they have great articles structured with subheadings to cover every aspect you can imagine (you'll need to register but it's free to do so). You'll also find lots of great information from medical colleges, patient associations, charities and the WHO.

One absolutely essential website to get to know right from the start is Geeky Medics (geekymedics.com). This has grown into a comprehensive resource covering just about everything a medical student needs to know, and is particularly helpful in the run-up to OSCEs. Other popular sites are listed in **Box 2.11**. And don't forget the legions of medical students who went before you: loads of them have shared their experiences through blogs and articles to help out their successors such as you. Some have even uploaded all of their notes and drawings, such as www.toddgreen.co.uk/medicine and happymednotes.blogspot.com. Aren't people nice!

A note of caution: you do need to be more discerning with websites than other learning resources, particularly if you came to them through Google, as there is a mind-boggling amount of incorrect, untrustworthy and outright biased information out there. Always check who publishes the website, who it is aimed at and what hidden agendas they might have when you are considering whether it is an appropriate resource for medical students. And definitely think twice before citing information in presentations or tutorials: no matter how easy-going your tutor is, they're not going to be impressed when your source turns out to be an article from the Mail Online's sidebar of shame.

**Box 2.11**

**Top websites for medical students**

- Geeky Medics (geekymedics.com)
- Oxford Medical Education (oxfordmedicaleducation.com)
- Almost a Doctor (almostadoctor.co.uk)
- NHS (nhs.uk)
- Medscape (medscape.com)
- Wikipedia (wikipedia.org)
- Patient (patient.info/patientplus)
- Anatomy Zone (anatomyzone.com)
- MedRevise (medrevise.co.uk)
- Medical student blogs

## 2.5.10 Cartoons

If you're a particularly visual learner, you'll be delighted to discover a whole world of educational medical illustrations, cartoons and comics. Many are of an incredibly high standard and are an absolute joy to study from (not all are free, unsurprisingly, given how much effort goes into them). Take a look at SketchyMedical, Medcomic and Kloss & Bruce to get you started, and if you want to go even further down the rabbit hole visit www.graphicmedicine.org. I would also recommend the cartoons (and books on *Surviving Medicine*) of Will Sloper (www.unicyclemedic.com) – a personal favourite for when you need some light relief and a good laugh at the occasional absurdity of medicine!

### 2.5.11 Summary

In this section, we have looked at some study resources to help you survive the preclinical years. These form the tools that allow you to build up your bricks of knowledge. The key points are:

- Use a wide variety of different resources to study.
- Give extra importance to lecture slides as they offer a guide to what's in your exams.
- Be open-minded and keep looking for new resources: there are fresh apps, websites, online tutorials and books emerging all the time.
- Study actively when watching online tutorials: don't just zone out and hope the information will stick somehow.
- Build your own resources such as flashcards, MCQs and quizzes. This is a great way to learn.
- Dip into question banks but go sparingly at this stage – you will rely heavily on them during later years so don't peak too early.

# 2.6 Essential skills: surviving the preclinical years without going insane

## 2.6.1 Manage your time effectively

Perhaps the greatest skill you can teach yourself in the early years of medical school is how to manage your time effectively. This can be very difficult to master, but will set you up superbly for the clinical years if you can manage it.

**TOP TIP**

Three important steps towards managing your time more effectively:
1. Take control of your time and make conscious decisions about how to spend it.
2. Ensure that studying and me-time are both represented and that you have struck a reasonable balance between the two.
3. Treat your time with respect by actually using slots in the way you intended and not blurring the boundaries between study and relaxation time.

The first step towards good time management is to recognise that you have control over your time and can actively choose how to spend it, as opposed to passively drifting wherever the tide takes you. Exert this control by dividing your time into slots for studying and for 'me-time' such as socialising, playing sports or relaxing. Slots can be any size and shape. For example, you have two hours free between lectures: you might designate this as study time and spend it in the library, or you might decide to take some me-time and go for a swim and get a coffee. Either option is absolutely fine – but the point is to make *a conscious decision* about how to spend those two hours instead of just standing around chatting after the lecture and seeing what happens. If you've actively decided to use that time for relaxing rather than studying, then by all means stand around and chat! Just as long as you have thought it through.

The second step is to ensure you strike a good balance between study time and me-time, and don't exclusively fill your slots with one or the other. You'll need to be honest with yourself and have some self-discipline: there are seven evenings in a week, can you really justify spending *all* of them playing PlayStation? I'd suggest three evenings of study time and four of me-time might be a better balance! Likewise those free slots in between lectures: if you hung out with your friends on Monday and Wednesday, then you should probably study on Tuesday and Thursday to balance it out. And yes, weekends are precious – believe me, I know that – but *surely* you can spare a few hours for studying? If you were too hung-over to do any work on Saturday, then perhaps Sunday is a good day to make up for it? The reverse is also true:

**You will rapidly burn out if you try to study every hour of every day, so make sure you properly offset your study time with some relaxation and non-medical time.**

> Never feel bad about taking time off from studying to relax, provided you have done enough work to justify it. Medical school is a very long game and it is absolutely essential that you pace yourself and set time aside to recharge your batteries. Do not let medicine take over your life, because it will if you're not careful!

**TOP TIP**

The third step is to view your time as a precious and finite resource which, once used up, cannot be got back. You should therefore treat it with respect by setting clear boundaries between study time and me-time and actually using these slots in the way you intended, rather than wasting them by accident. In other words, if you've set aside some study time, then give it your full attention and **use it to study**, not to text your friends, play pool or watch Love Island. And if you've set aside an evening to relax, then find something nice to do and **relax** – don't half-heartedly flick through PassMedicine questions in front of the TV just to make yourself feel like you are doing something. This blurring of the boundaries between study time and me-time is inefficient and can be very damaging to morale as it makes you constantly feel like you're not really achieving anything. A wise Scotsman once told me: "You cannae ride two bikes with one arse". He's right. Make sure your arse is on one bike at a time and you'll find it a lot easier to travel forwards.

## 2.6.2 Get into good routines and habits

In the early stages of medical school, it can be very tempting to just take each day as it comes: to wake up in the morning, see what's on your timetable, decide what you feel like attending and then go with the flow from there. This approach is understandable, particularly when you have a busy social schedule and are adjusting to your new life as a student living away from home. There's so much going on, it can feel very restrictive to make too many plans or attempt to think too far ahead.

I would, however, encourage you to reframe this thinking: instead of viewing each day in isolation, try to think of medical school as one long and continuous process, in which the individual days add up to form a much larger whole. This means there is huge value in building good routines and habits into your day because, however small they seem on their own, those good habits will add up and multiply with every day that you repeat them, delivering huge payoffs over the longer term.

I came to this conclusion while commuting an hour each way to medical school every day on the London Underground. This initially felt like a grind, but turned out to be a blessing in disguise as it gave me two hours per day of protected study time (forget sitting in the library – some of my best revision was done standing up with my face pressed into a stranger's sweaty armpit). Looking back, this was hugely beneficial for me and probably a significant factor in my success.

**Your days are full of these little timeslots when you might otherwise not be doing anything useful – particularly in the mornings and early evenings. Do not just ignore them: look for them, carve them out and do your best to maximise them day in, day out, week after week.**

Now, I'm not suggesting you move out of town and commute back in, but ask yourself honestly: how difficult would it really be to carve out an hour of study time each morning before going into university? Or between getting home and going out in the evening? For example, let's say your lectures usually finish at 5 p.m. on a Tuesday and you go to the gym at 7 p.m., after which you eat dinner and then are always too tired to do any work. That's fair enough – you can't force yourself to work when your brain won't comply! But consider that slot beforehand: instead of just killing time until 7, let's say you get home by 5.30, knuckle down and do one hour of good, efficient studying before heading off to the gym.

That hour might not sound like very much, but if you can carve out an extra hour like this every weekday when you might otherwise not have bothered: hey, that's five hours a week of extra study time you just bagged yourself. And five hours a week adds up to 20 hours a month, which adds up to 240 hours a year. That's ten entire days' worth of extra study time over the year, all from building just one measly extra hour into your daily routine!

**TOP TIP**

Try to carve out one extra hour of study time each day, such as by getting out of bed earlier in the morning and doing some reading over breakfast, or by working for an hour before going out for the evening. These seemingly small amounts will really add up over the months and years.

There are loads of other great habits you can get into from day one of medical school, as shown in **Box 2.12**. These will all help you to study more effectively, get information to stick in your brain better and – above all – to look after yourself and stay sane over the next few years!

**Great habits to improve your studying and keep yourself sane at medical school**

Box 2.12

- Minimise distractions: whenever you are studying, **put your phone away**, turn off notifications on your laptop, and ensure you can concentrate fully on whatever you're doing.
- Exercise and eat healthily: looking after your body will help keep your mind sharp.
- Plan ahead: look at your timetable at the start of each week and make a sensible plan for when and how you are going to study. Stick to it as best you can!
- Be honest and realistic: don't set overly ambitious targets which you are never going to achieve, as this will just stress you out.
- Pat yourself on the back when you've had a good study session and achieved your goals. Accept there will always be more you could have done and don't get stressed out by this.
- Vary your study techniques and resources to keep things fresh.
- Have a good filing system and hang onto helpful resources you find. You'll want to use them again in later years so make sure you can find them again.
- Maintain your favourite hobbies and activities: do not let medical school take over your life!
- Do non-medical things with non-medics: living in the bubble can be stifling, so make sure to stick your head outside for fresh air.
- Don't be ruled by FOMO (fear of missing out): there will *always* be some sort of social event going on somewhere – you simply can't do everything and some amount of sacrifice is sadly unavoidable!

## 2.6.3 Be an active studier

Whatever topic, technique and resources you are using, you should always try to study ***actively***. This means ***doing stuff*** instead of zoning out, ***engaging your brain*** instead of switching off and ***keeping yourself involved*** with the topic at hand instead of letting it simply wash over you and vainly hoping something will stick. See ***Table 2.8*** for some examples of how you can go about this. A little self-awareness is important: it's normal to zone out for little periods here and there, but try to recognise when it's happening, take a break then kick yourself back into gear. Don't just write off entire sessions by being passive because you will find it very hard to retain information this way, and then your time has been wasted.

**Table 2.8: Examples of active versus passive studying**

| Activity | Passive studier | Active studier |
|---|---|---|
| **Attending a lecture on the physiology of the cardiac cycle** | Sits there listening, trying to concentrate but soon loses interest and starts daydreaming | Reads up in advance, brings a copy of the slides, annotates them, does drawings, looks up things they are unsure about, asks questions at the end, returns to their notes later to re-read and edit them |
| **Attending a dissection room session on abdominal anatomy** | Watches and listens to the anatomy demonstrators and other students, but does not get involved unless forced to | Reads up in advance, gets hands-on with the cadavers, considers clinical implications of the anatomy, asks questions throughout, makes notes and consolidates learning afterwards |
| **Attending a small-group tutorial on microbiology** | Shows up, listens, leaves | Reads up in advance, makes notes while others are talking, takes part in discussions and demonstrations, asks questions, helps others out, reviews notes afterwards, tests themselves the next day, builds new-found knowledge into notes, mind maps and flashcards |

## 2.6.4 Love the fluff

Before starting medical school, I thought fluff was just something you found in your belly button at the end of a long day. But I quickly learned that it is disparaging slang used by medical students for topics like ethics, law, professionalism, statistics, sociology and epidemiology. In other words: the stuff you get taught which **isn't** straight clinical and scientific material like anatomy and physiology.

I observed a strong tendency among med students to sneer at the fluff in the early years – to look down their noses at it and deem it less worthy of their time and effort than other, 'proper' subjects (it doesn't help that these topics suffer dreadfully from a branding problem: at my med school, the official name for these parts of the course was 'Community and Population Health/Personal and Professional Development', or CPH/PPD for short. With a name as catchy as that, it's no wonder people called it fluff).

Now, me, I'm a touchy-feely, slipper-wearing old fart who finds ethics and law genuinely interesting. But even if you absolutely hate these topics, I urge you **not** to make the mistake of neglecting them during your preclinical years. This is a common trap which I observed many, many students fall into.

Six reasons to love the 'fluff': ethics, professionalism, law, statistics, etc.
1. Comes up often in exams.
2. Topics are predictable.
3. Marks are easy to get with a little work.
4. Marks are easy to lose without a little work.
5. Answers can be easily structured.
6. You will need this knowledge throughout medical school and beyond.

**KEY POINT**

Neglecting the fluff is a mistake because these topics are **extremely** likely to come up in exams (particularly post-Harold Shipman, when medical schools have been under pressure to produce ethical, professional and compassionate doctors). And when they do come up, they tend to be easy marks because the topics are fairly predictable, so you know what to expect. Take ethics and law, for example: you can virtually guarantee that one of euthanasia/assisted dying, abortion, DNARs and healthcare rationing will come up. It would be utterly crazy to go into exams without a solid knowledge of these subjects, yet that is what countless medical students seem to do time and again, year after year.

The other great thing about medical ethics is that answers are easy to structure: let's say you are asked to write a short essay question, or asked for an ethical analysis in an OSCE, you can just reach immediately for the four pillars of autonomy, non-maleficence, beneficence and justice (**Figure 2.10**). Go through each of these in turn, say something vaguely sensible

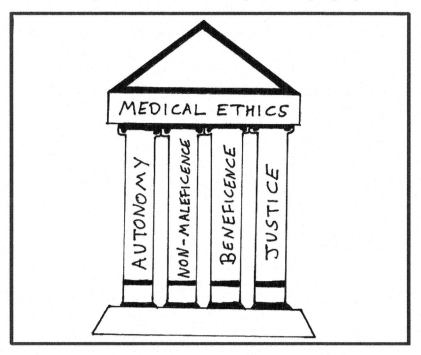

**Figure 2.10: The four pillars of medical ethics.** As an absolute minimum, you should know these off by heart and be able to use them as a framework to structure an answer or provide an ethical analysis in an OSCE. Neglect 'fluff' topics like this at your peril!

for each one, and you are basically guaranteed to get a passable mark and perhaps even a very good one. If you can't even recall the four pillars you are at a massive disadvantage before you even start. Essay questions tend to carry lots of marks so there is a lot to lose if you crash and burn. Get a multiple choice anatomy question wrong, by contrast, and you have only dropped one mark.

The final reason to take the fluff seriously is that, in my experience, it tended to come up consistently in exams and OSCEs throughout medical school, despite being mostly taught at the beginning. This is in contrast to clinical topics, where exams tended to stick more closely to material we had been taught in the preceding year only. What's more, in final year you'll have to take the Situational Judgement Test, which is a very important national exam dedicated entirely to fluff. So there really is no getting away from it – put some time and effort into these topics in the early days and you will reap the dividends later on.

## 2.6.5 Maximising lectures

Like a moth to a flame, as an older student I always found myself inexorably drawn to the front of the lecture theatre. Life down there is so civilised for us old folk: you can read the slides without having to squint, you can ask questions without needing to shout, and you can hear the lecturer clearly without your hearing aids. It's bliss. From there, if you turn around and look back, you can see only the backs of everyone's laptops: row after row of Apples and HPs gleaming through the half-light, with pairs of eyes poking out over the top. 'How studious everyone looks!' I thought to myself, safe in the assumption that they were busily typing notes, annotating slides and cross-referencing the material against other sources.

Imagine my shock, therefore, when one day I found myself sitting right at the back of the lecture theatre (heaven knows what I was doing back there – having an absence seizure, perhaps) and got to see the other side of the laptop screens. I witnessed an astonishing array of electronic activity – everything from YouTube, WhatsApp and Facebook to live sport, online shopping, games and puzzles – while the lecturer obliviously trundled on about mitosis and the cell cycle. It absolutely blew my mind.

Now don't get me wrong – I enjoy a YouTube binge as much as the next person – but doing this sort of thing in lectures is an epic waste of your time and a poor study strategy. Because no matter how dull the session turns out to be, you have already made the decision to attend it and are therefore investing a chunk of your precious time into it. So you owe it to yourself to try to extract something educational from that lecture, no matter how small, otherwise the entire hour was wasted and you will never get it back. If you want to watch cat videos and play Candy Crush for an hour then go for it – but make a conscious decision to do so, then just do it at home and save yourself the hassle of showing up!

Hopefully it won't come to this as your lectures will be really interesting and enjoyable. Here's how you can ensure you extract the most from any lecture you attend:

**Table 2.9: How to get the most out of lectures**

| **Beforehand** | • Look at the slides and have a quick read around the subject |
| | • Bring the slides with you, either on paper or electronically |
| | • Make sure you have water, coffee, snacks or whatever you need to keep yourself awake and engaged |
| **During** | • Listen actively, keeping your brain engaged |
| | • Make lots of notes, either on paper or your computer (programs like Evernote and OneNote allow you to annotate the lecturers' slides) |
| | • Put your phone away and silence notifications on your laptop |
| | • Quickly look up things you don't understand, or make a list of things to look up later |
| | • If you are flagging, allow yourself a short mental time out then rejoin the action; don't just give up and zone out completely |
| | • Consider sitting closer to the front if you are finding yourself getting too distracted |
| **After** | • Re-read your notes and the slides while fresh in your mind |
| | • Type them up if handwritten, editing them as you do so |
| | • Consider whether any parts could be rewritten as a table, mind map or diagram |
| | • Incorporate all of this material into your existing notes and study resources such as flashcards |

Unfortunately, despite all your best efforts, some lectures will be boring and you'll struggle to pay attention. When this does happen, challenge yourself to find at least **three things** you can learn from the lecture. This is a very achievable target! If the rest of it truly sucks then you can use the remaining time to discreetly look these three things up in other sources and start writing your own notes on them. And if you really find it hard to pay attention in lectures then why not try sitting closer to the front? Trust me, everything is better down there!

Challenge yourself to learn at least three things from any lecture you attend. Test yourself after to ensure you can recall your three facts.

## 2.6.6 Maximising PBL and tutorials

Problem-based learning (PBL), or problem-based eating as I prefer to call it, is medical school speak for getting students to work through scenarios together in small groups whilst eating a mega-ton of snacks. As an educational strategy it has its pros and cons (see *Table 2.10*), but as a way to put on a stone in your first month of university it really is hard to beat.

PBL is a relatively modern approach to teaching medicine, having debuted in the UK in 1984. The general principle is to make learning more interactive, self-directed and team-based, and to move away from everything being taught by lecture. PBL usually takes the form of three tutorials held over the week, typically Monday, Wednesday and Friday, during which you'll work your way through a clinical case that aligns with whatever topic you are learning about that week: diabetes, for example

**Table 2.10: The pros and cons of problem-based learning (PBL)**

| Pros | Cons |
|---|---|
| • Sociable, fun way to learn | • Potential for personality clashes and fallouts |
| • Your learning can be enhanced by other students | • Your learning can be hindered by other students |
| • Safe space to share ideas | • The team will often generate wrong ideas and misinformation – PBL relies on the tutor to correct these |
| • Promotes teamwork which is good preparation for being a doctor | • Requires self-motivation to cover all the topics: this suits some people better than others |
| • Gives you some control over your workload | |
| • Forces you to engage actively with a subject, as opposed to lectures where you are passively absorbing information | • Monday tutorials can be annoying when you are expected to brainstorm a topic you know nothing about yet |
| • Makes lectures feel more relevant and interesting when you have already brainstormed that topic in a tutorial | • Inefficiency: you can waste time and effort generating LOBs which aren't relevant |
| • Develops your research and critical appraisal skills | • Tutorials can *really* drag on, especially if you cover the material quickly |
| • Injects variety into your week | • Feels patronising to have your timetable and LOBs 'hidden' from you until after the Monday tutorial |
| • Emphasis on problem solving helps you start to think like a doctor | |

**Table 2.11: The typical weekly cycle of PBL tutorials.** The rest of the week comprises lectures, seminars, dissection, clinical and communication skills and any other activities which build on the topics and themes set during PBL. Please note: the specifics will vary between medical schools.

| Monday Tutorial | Wednesday Tutorial | Friday Tutorial |
|---|---|---|
| • Wrap up last week's case<br><br>• Meet a new virtual patient and learn about their presenting complaint; this will set the tone and topics for the week<br><br>• Brainstorm ideas for what is wrong with the patient and generate LOBs for the week<br><br>• Receive your week's timetable at the end, which tells you which lectures and other sessions to expect | • Work through Monday's LOBs as a group, ensuring everyone understands all the material<br><br>• Find out what happened next in the case, discuss it and generate more LOBs | • Work through Wednesday's LOBs as a group<br><br>• Find out what happened next in the case, discuss it and generate more LOBs for the weekend |

(see *Table 2.11*). The catch is that you don't know what the topic is to begin with, so you might start the Monday tutorial faced with a patient who has weight loss, polyuria and excessive thirst – you'll initially have no clue what's going on but you'll brainstorm a load of possible causes and generate your own LOBs to go away and study. A tutor facilitates the discussion and provides some gentle guidance without giving too much away. That's PBL in a nutshell: if you're really interested you can read more here.[3]

Some medical schools, like mine, use a lot of PBL, others use a small amount and others don't use it at all. Some use variations like case-based learning or enquiry-based learning. Whatever. For the purposes of our discussion, let's talk in general terms about any type of small-group tutorial where you and your peers are given scenarios or clinical cases to work through as a team. With snacks, obvs.

When any new group of people is formed, there will be a natural period of adjustment at the start while people settle on their roles: the extrovert who constantly dominates discussion, the introvert who rarely makes a peep, the passive aggressive one who guns down everyone else's ideas while offering none of their own, and the wannabe comedian who turns everything into a knob joke.

3 *BMJ* 2003;326:328

**Try not to get drawn into personality contests or let certain people take over: you'll find the group functions best when everyone gets along, respects and listens to each other.**

And the better the group functions, the more you will learn which – let's not forget – is the entire aim of the exercise. (And to eat snacks. Did I mention the snacks?)

Tutorials are a fantastic opportunity to study with your course mates, learn from each other, calibrate your knowledge and swap ideas, resources and techniques. You also get incredible insights to the way other people think, strategise and solve problems. If someone else impresses you – try to learn from them and emulate them. If you think they're useless – do the opposite! I found this a very powerful strategy in my first year: it was clear who the knowledgeable and hard-working students were in my groups, so I made an extra effort to listen when they spoke and be influenced by their ideas. This worked well for me and I would encourage you to do the same.

**TOP TIP**

Force yourself out of your comfort zone and take an active role in group discussions. You will learn much more this way!

Another super-important thing about tutorials is that they provide an opportunity to test and challenge yourself by explaining ideas and concepts to the group. Take an active role in discussions, put forward your own thoughts and stand up and draw things on the whiteboard whenever you get the opportunity. You will get things wrong and make mistakes – that is absolutely fine – but you will learn *infinitely* more than if you just stay silent in the corner. This requires the self-motivation to drag yourself outside your comfort zone, but it will be worth it in the end. And trust me, tutorials are a much nicer, safer environment to present an X-ray, for example, than the morning trauma and orthopaedics meeting when the scary-ass consultant – fresh from aggressively bollocking his registrar for missing the fracture – asks you, the medical student, to stand up and point it out to a whole room full of people. Gulp.

Here are some other ways you can make the most of PBLs and other small-group tutorials:

- Put in some work beforehand so you can make useful contributions.
- Adopt a 'no notes' approach: have your notes in the room but *do not* look at them when you are presenting an idea or during the discussions. This gives you the chance to truly test your *knowledge*, rather than your ability to read off a page.

- Don't be scared to make mistakes – you can learn a lot by doing so.
- Be ready to explain any of the LOBs if called upon, as opposed to just working on a few you like the look of and ignoring the rest.
- Rehearse the information in your head beforehand and have an idea of how you would explain it accurately and concisely to the rest of the group if called upon.
- Use structured frameworks for discussion (see below).
- Listen to other people when they are talking.
- Ask questions if you don't understand something.
- Jot down any great ideas, resources or study strategies you come across.
- Look over your notes afterwards to consolidate your knowledge.

Structured frameworks really come into their own in PBL because they provide direction and focus to the discussion and ensure that everyone can follow it. We have already talked about Dr Deac Pimp as a way to study a particular disease (see **Section 2.4.6**), but what about in tutorials when you are given a case to work through and you don't yet know what the disease or problem is?

Let's use the example of a patient presenting with shortness of breath – a classic high-yield topic. Rather than everyone just shouting out random diseases like 'asthma' or 'heart attack', you should try as a group to work through it in a systematic fashion. Here are two different ways to do that:

## 1. Group by body system

Write the following headings on the board (these are just examples, you can do any systems you think are relevant, in any order):

- Cardiovascular
- Respiratory
- Haematological
- Psychological
- Musculoskeletal

Then work through these systems one by one, as a team, with people taking it in turns to suggest conditions which could cause shortness of breath. For example:

- Cardiovascular: myocardial infarction, heart failure, aortic dissection
- Respiratory: asthma, COPD, pulmonary embolism, inhaled foreign body
- Haematological: anaemia, leukaemia

- Psychological: anxiety, panic attacks
- Musculoskeletal: obesity, chest wall deformities

Approaches like this not only improve the structure and quality of the discussion, but also help you start to develop the logical, structured thinking pattern you will need as a doctor. After all, patients don't present with a disease written on their forehead: they present with a bunch of symptoms, and it is up to you to work out what's causing them. This is a great way to start doing that!

## 2.  Surgical sieve

A surgical sieve is essentially a thought process which provides an even more structured approach to thinking about differential diagnoses. You'll come across loads of different 'sieve' mnemonics which you can use, based on your preference. I always liked **VITAMIN CDEF**, which goes like this:

- **V** = vascular
- **I** = infective/inflammatory
- **T** = traumatic
- **A** = autoimmune
- **M** = metabolic
- **I** = iatrogenic (fancy word for side-effects/complications of medical treatments)
- **N** = neoplastic (fancy word for cancer)
- **C** = congenital
- **D** = degenerative
- **E** = endocrine
- **F** = functional (fancy word for not having any organic/physical cause)

So, sticking with the shortness of breath example, you might come up with the following:

- Vascular: myocardial infarction, pulmonary embolism, aortic dissection, arrhythmias
- Infective/inflammatory: pneumonia, sepsis, anaphylaxis, asthma
- Traumatic: chest injury, pneumothorax
- Autoimmune: sarcoidosis
- Metabolic: diabetic ketoacidosis, anaemia

- Iatrogenic: medication side-effect such as pulmonary fibrosis from long-term methotrexate or amiodarone use
- Neoplastic: lung cancer, upper airway tumours
- Congenital: chest wall deformities such as scoliosis
- Degenerative: heart failure, COPD
- Endocrine: hypothyroidism
- Functional: anxiety, panic attacks

The advantage of surgical sieves is they are very comprehensive, forcing you to cover things you might not otherwise think of. These will be extremely helpful throughout your medical career, so tutorials are a great place to start using them. Hopefully now you know what to expect and are equipped to hit the ground running from tutorial number one!

## 2.6.7 Maximising self-directed learning

Depending on the vibe of your med school, they will give you a certain amount of free time during the preclinical years for self-directed learning (SDL). Half or whole days off present a golden opportunity to get some great studying done, yet a lot of students struggle to make the most of them. Many times, a free afternoon begins with good intentions but ends up asleep face down in a textbook or worse, in the pub (don't get me wrong: I was rarely one to decline the chance for a pint, but try to get some good work done before you go and avoid making a habit of it!).

To truly make the most of SDL time, you will need to bring together all the skills we have covered so far, particularly time management and using a range of different techniques and resources. But we also need to introduce an extremely important new concept known as Parkinson's law. Named after historian Cyril Northcote Parkinson (no relation to James Parkinson, for whom the disease is named), this law is usually defined as:

> **"Work expands to fill the time available for its completion."**

Or, to put it another way: if I gave you a deadline of three weeks to write an essay, you would almost certainly take three weeks to write that essay and submit it on the final day. If I gave you a deadline of three hours to write an essay, you would have that essay miraculously written in three hours. Two very different time periods, yet the **exact same endpoint** is reached. The three-hour deadline was therefore much more efficient for maximising output!

Parkinson's law essentially articulates what we all know in our hearts to be true: that we humans are inherently inefficient and will faff around and procrastinate unless we are given clear targets and deadlines. For big chunks of SDL time, therefore, you need to turn Parkinson's law to your advantage by setting yourself a series of tasks with allocated time slots. The law dictates that you will get through these tasks within their deadlines, achieving a lot in the process. On the other hand, if you set yourself a couple of small, unambitious tasks or no tasks at all, you will **still fill the exact same amount of time** but without achieving nearly as much.

**KEY POINT**

Parkinson's law suggests that work will take up as much time as you have available for it. Turn this to your advantage by assigning deadlines to tasks, so you can get through more work in the same amount of time.

With this concept in mind, let's introduce my three-phase strategy for maximising your SDL sessions (**Figure 2.11**). First you need to **plan** them with a strong focus on clear targets and efficient time management, then you need to **execute** that plan properly. The final phase is to **consolidate** and reinforce your learning afterwards to ensure the information sticks. You can adapt this approach to any topic and any substantial time slot you have available for SDL, and hopefully you will find you start achieving more in the hours you have available.

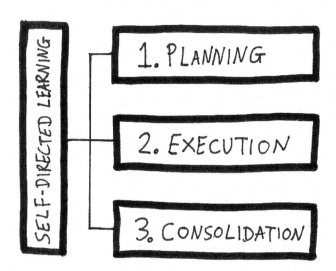

**Figure 2.11: A three-phase strategy for maximising your SDL time.**

**SDL phase 1: Planning**

Do this at the beginning of your study session or the night before.
Ensure your plan is realistic, achievable and won't stress you out!
1. Pick your topics based on lecture slides and your weekly LOBs.
2. Break them into chunks.
3. Decide which chunks to cover in that session and which can wait.
4. Decide how much time to spend on each.
5. Choose your techniques.
6. Choose your resources.
7. Decide how you will test your new-found knowledge.

Box 2.13

**SDL phase 2: Execution**

1. Don't procrastinate: start on time and work steadily through the tasks and deadlines you have set yourself.
2. Take regular breaks.
3. Eat well and keep hydrated.
4. Get your work done in the time you set aside for it.
5. Go do something else!

Box 2.14

**SDL phase 3: Consolidation**

This is every bit as crucial as the studying itself: without it, the new-found knowledge will simply fade from your brain over time.
1. Look back over your notes at the first opportunity.
2. Edit and condense them, adding in mind maps, drawings, tables and flashcards.
3. Keep track of topics you *didn't* cover yet (very important!).
4. Keep reviewing your notes and testing yourself, paying close attention to things you keep getting wrong.
5. Review the topic a few weeks later in study group.

Box 2.15

Let's work through an example, based on a real-life week I had at medical school. The topic is the eye and you are planning how to spend the free Tuesday morning you've been given for SDL. You have the following LOBs to cover:

- Structure and function of the eye and the extraocular muscles
- Neural pathways involved in vision
- Cataracts
- Glaucoma

Here's how you might go about tackling this:

## Phase 1: Planning

- Allow yourself one hour on Monday night to plan your SDL session.
- Skim through the lecture slides to establish how complex these topics are.
- These four LOBs would be too much for a single morning so you will have to prioritise: do this with your timetable in mind, so that your SDL aligns with your formal teaching.
- In this case, let's say you decide to focus on the structure and function of the eye plus glaucoma, and leave the other topics until later.
- Devise a realistic, achievable plan for your SDL session: see **Table 2.12** for a worked example and **Table 2.13** for a blank template.

## Phase 2: Execution

- Start promptly and stick to your plan, taking breaks to stretch your legs, go to the toilet and get coffee.
- Stay cool if you don't get through everything in the time allocated – just do your best and move on to the next task when time is finished. Don't let a single task take over the whole morning.
- Remember the key concept of spiral learning from **Chapter 1**: you are just laying the foundations, so it is better to cover all your topics in basic detail than to go into immense depth on just one.
- Jot down anything you don't understand so you can ask the lecturer or bring it up in PBL.
- Finish on time and go for lunch and a catch-up with your friends!

## Phase 3: Consolidation

- Look back at your notes over breakfast on Wednesday.
- Present your knowledge in your PBL tutorial.
- Implement your testing strategies whenever you get a chance. These can be in short bursts; you don't need to set hours aside for this.
- Remember the things you **didn't** get around to yet – hopefully you get a chance later in the week, otherwise try to make time on the weekend so you don't fall behind.
- Edit your notes once the week's teaching is finished, including making a one-page summary of everything you need to know about the eye.
- Review your notes again soon and go over the whole subject again in study group a month later to make sure you don't forget it.

**Table 2.12: Example of how you might spend a morning of SDL in the library studying the eye, using some of the techniques and resources we have learned so far**

| Time | Topic | Techniques | Resources | Testing strategies |
|---|---|---|---|---|
| 9.00–10.00 | Anatomy: Structure of the eye | • Draw a colourful picture of an eye in cross-section<br>• Make brief notes around the side about the key structures<br>• Add arrows to sketch out the flow of aqueous humour | • Anatomy textbook<br>• Anatomy app<br>• Premade anatomy flashcards | • Redraw the eye from memory<br>• Practise the flashcards<br>• Attempt some questions from the anatomy textbook<br>• Take an active role in the dissection session and see how much you remember |
| 10.15–11.15 | Physiology: Function of the eye | • Watch an online video tutorial on visual physiology<br>• Make a table summarising the key points<br>• Write 5 quiz questions based on your table | • Lecture slides<br>• YouTube tutorials<br>• Physiology textbook | • Fill the table in from memory<br>• Attempt your quiz questions<br>• Take the lead in explaining this topic in PBL, without looking at your notes |
| 11.30–12.30 | Pathology: Glaucoma | • Start filling out a Dr Deac Pimp on glaucoma (you probably won't finish it in an hour but that's fine)<br>• Make a mind map to go with it | • Lecture slides<br>• Basic ophthalmology book (e.g. *At a Glance*)<br>• BMJ Best Practice or UpToDate<br>• Websites (e.g. glaucoma charities and associations) | • Redraw the mind map from memory<br>• Make your own electronic flashcards<br>• Attempt some MCQs from an online question bank |

Table 2.13: Blank template for planning any SDL session

| Time | Topic | Techniques | Resources | Testing strategies |
|------|-------|------------|-----------|--------------------|
|      |       |            |           |                    |
|      |       |            |           |                    |
|      |       |            |           |                    |

## 2.6.8 Summary

In this section, we have looked at some of the essential skills needed to do well in your preclinical years without going insane. The key points are:

- Manage your time effectively by taking control of it, finding a healthy balance between work time and me-time, and using your time in the way you intended without blurring the boundaries between study and relaxation.
- Never feel bad about taking time for yourself, as long as you have done enough studying to justify it.
- Med school is a very long game: get into good routines and habits from day one and these will serve you well over the years.
- Study actively and engage with the subject: if you just zone out you are essentially wasting your time.
- Take the 'fluff' seriously: it's interesting, important and worth a lot of marks.
- Maximise lectures by preparing in advance, writing lots of notes and going over them afterwards. Try to learn at least three things from any lecture you attend.
- Maximise PBL and small-group tutorials by putting in some work beforehand and taking an active role in discussions.
- Maximise SDL time by using a three-pronged approach: planning, execution and consolidation.
- Turn Parkinson's law to your advantage by setting yourself clear tasks and deadlines when you have a large chunk of free time for SDL.

# 2.7 Clinical and communication skills: level I

Assuming your brain hasn't exploded yet, I'd like to introduce you to another essential strand of your medical education: clinical and communication skills (and if it has exploded, well, at least your friends can learn how to do a fun neurological examination on you). These are the classes where they teach you how to do proper doctor-y stuff like ask a patient what's wrong with them, listen to their heart, look in their ears and put your finger up their bum. Or, to use the boring technical terms: take a history, perform a cardiovascular examination, practise otoscopy and carry out a *per rectum* (PR) examination.

I found clinical and communication skills a real highlight of my early years at medical school because they're hands-on, fun, interactive and involve actually **doing** stuff. There's also the fact that you get to start imagining yourself being a doctor for the first time – it'll still seem scary and far off, but at least you'll feel like you're finally in the ballpark. I enjoyed clinical skills so much I became a peer tutor in my later years of medical school and a clinical skills lead in FY1. Much better than hanging out with the cadavers in the basement, in my humble opinion!

The list of skills you need to learn as a medical student is enormous: there's examinations for every system and joint in the body, plus loads of different history structures and practical procedures ranging from blood taking to inserting catheters. And once the teaching starts, they'll come thick and fast: you'll probably be expected to learn a new skill every one or two weeks. By my count, I had to learn around 45 different practical skills and ten clinical histories in my first two years of medical school, and that's a conservative estimate.

How are you possibly going to keep up with this, on top of all the academic stuff you're supposed to learn? By taking a deep breath, keeping calm and doing the following:

## 2.7.1 Double down on structured frameworks and mnemonics

The only way you are **ever** going to survive the onslaught of clinical and communication skills is to learn repetitive formulae which you can apply to any and every situation. It's bonkers to try to learn 45 different skills from scratch – you're much better to look for the similarities, focus on learning some general principles and then build each new skill onto that common scaffolding. This is a lot more efficient and takes up less brain space!

*Figure 2.12* has the three key templates you need to know to get started. WIPER is a series of steps to follow **before** performing any examination on a patient. They're essential to good medical practice, respecting the patient's autonomy and facilitating a smooth and competent examination. You will also pick up a lot of marks in OSCEs for completing these basic steps, and drop a lot of marks by not doing so. Imagine if you were the patient and a doctor came and started poking you without introducing themselves, telling you what they were doing or washing their hands. You'd be pretty pissed off and rightly so!

If WIPER was the starter, IPPA is the main course: these are the steps you follow **during** any medical examination, to detect clinical signs that tell you what is going on with the patient. And WaTER is the dessert: your closing steps to round off your examination before you leave the room.

This, right here, is a beautiful point in your medical education. Stop, sniff the air and savour it. Because without even realising it you have just learned the basics of performing **absolutely any** clinical examination and are now well on the way to becoming a doctor. Don't believe me? Let's recap: WIPER ➔ IPPA ➔ WaTER. Repeat: WIPER ➔ IPPA ➔ WaTER.

Now imagine I asked you to go and examine a patient's abdomen. Without knowing **anything** about abdominal examination, you would now do the following:

1. Wash your hands, introduce yourself, get informed consent, ask if the patient has any pain, expose their abdomen and position them on the bed.

2. Inspect their abdomen, feel their abdomen, tap their abdomen and listen to their abdomen.

3. Wash your hands, thank the patient, ensure they are comfortable and report your findings.

And there you have it – the essentials of an abdominal examination! Now of course this isn't perfect, there is still plenty of fine-tuning required, but it's an excellent start and might even be good enough to pass a first-year OSCE station.

*Box 2.16* has some more generic structures you will need to learn for clinical and communication skills (they don't all have catchy mnemonics I'm afraid!). These might not all be familiar to you yet, but believe me, at some point you are going to need to learn them off by heart, inside out, back to front and upside down.

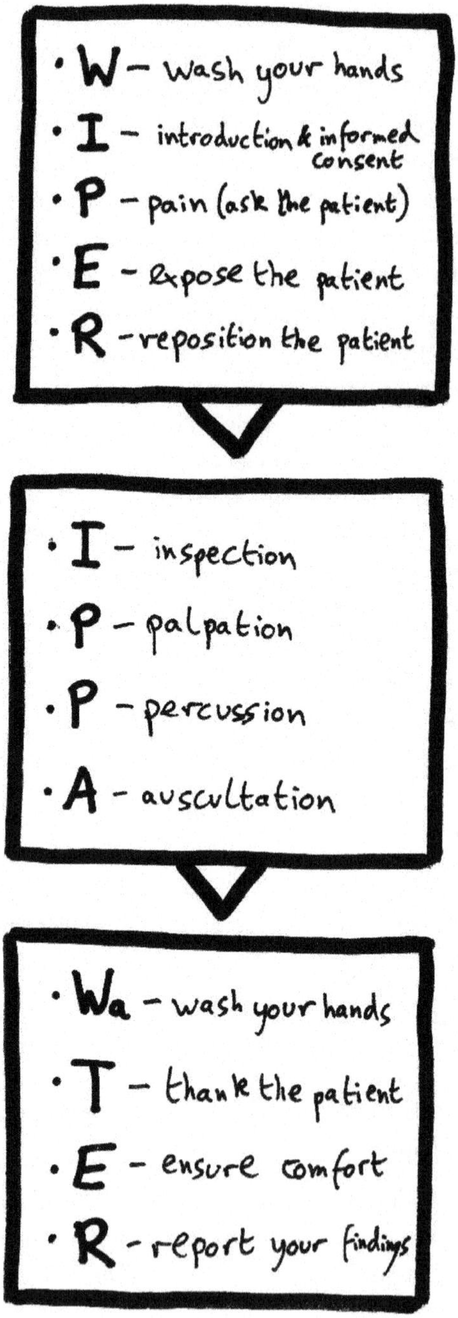

Figure 2.12: A generic framework you can apply to any clinical examination, in real life or OSCEs. Once you've got this down pat, you can start to adapt it to whichever examination you are doing (see *Section 2.7.3*).

- **W** – wash your hands
- **I** – introduction & informed consent
- **P** – pain (ask the patient)
- **E** – expose the patient
- **R** – reposition the patient

- **I** – inspection
- **P** – palpation
- **P** – percussion
- **A** – auscultation

- **Wa** – wash your hands
- **T** – thank the patient
- **E** – ensure comfort
- **R** – report your findings

**More structured frameworks for clinical and communication skills**

Box 2.16

**Basic clinical history:**
Presenting complaint
History of the presenting complaint
Past medical and surgical history
Drug history
Family history
Social history

**Pain history:** SOCRATES
**S**ite
**O**nset
**C**haracter
**R**adiation
**A**ssociated symptoms
**T**iming
**E**xacerbating and relieving factors
**S**everity
**ICE:** (demonstrate listening skills and empathy by exploring the patient's ...)
**I**deas
**C**oncerns
**E**xpectations

**Musculoskeletal examinations:**
Look
Feel
Move (active, passive and resisted)
Special tests

**Describing a lump: 4 Ss, 4 Ts and 4 Cs**

| | | |
|---|---|---|
| Site | Temperature | Consistency |
| Size | Tenderness | Contour |
| Shape | Tethering | Colour |
| Skin changes | Transillumination | Cough |

**Neurological examination:** I, Tony Power, Can See Red:
**I**nspection
**T**one
**P**ower
**C**oordination
**S**ensation
**R**eflexes

Why am I so obsessed with these structured approaches? Because you, me and everyone else, we are **fallible human beings**. We make mistakes. We get flustered. We say stupid things. And above all – **we forget stuff**.

> **In the heat of bedside teaching, or in an OSCE station, I absolutely guarantee your brain will desert you at crucial moments, leaving you unsure where you are up to in your history or examination. With a clear structure to fall back on, you can pause, mentally run through the steps and figure out exactly what you still have left to do.**

Without a structure, you can start to flounder, helplessly grasping at mental straws. If this happens in an OSCE, heaven help you, you risk unravelling before the examiner's eyes, haemorrhaging marks and plunging into a downward spiral of doom. This is something we desperately want to avoid, so better get learning those structures!

## 2.7.2 Work anatomically

Alongside mnemonics, another important method for approaching clinical examination is to work in a predetermined anatomical order. You open with a general inspection from the end of the bed, then move to the patient's hands, then work your way up to the arms, then the face, then down to the neck, then the chest and/or back, then the abdomen and finally to the legs (**Figure 2.13**). At each stage, pause for a second and ask yourself: do I need to do anything here? If so, do whichever bits of IPPA are relevant. We'll work through an example in **Section 2.7.3**.

This order of steps is a widely accepted convention in medicine, so you will need to get to grips with it if you want to fit in and look the part! It's actually really helpful when you are first learning these examinations because it means that even if you forget to do certain things – which you inevitably will – at least you'll know where to go to next and can keep moving through the examination in an orderly fashion rather than tripping up and grinding to a halt. And if you remember something later, you can always come back and do it at the end.

Just to be clear: the anatomical approach doesn't work for every clinical skill, but it does cover the big three of cardiovascular, respiratory and abdominal examination. These are absolutely core skills, virtually guaranteed to come up in OSCEs, so they are well worth putting some effort into!

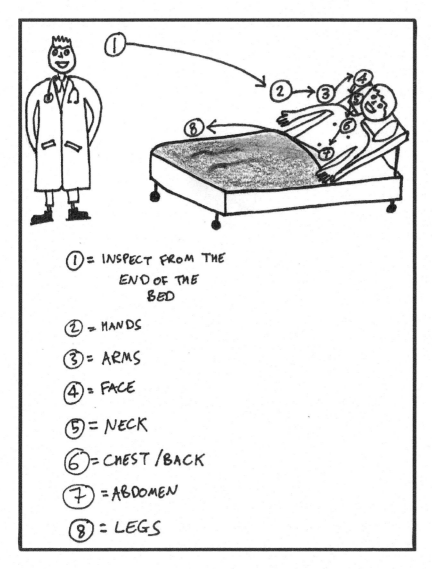

① = INSPECT FROM THE
        END OF THE
            BED

② = HANDS

③ = ARMS

④ = FACE

⑤ = NECK

⑥ = CHEST /BACK

⑦ = ABDOMEN

⑧ = LEGS

**Figure 2.13: How to work anatomically when examining a patient.** This order is a widely accepted convention in medicine, and will help you to keep track of where you are up to in your examination.

## 2.7.3 Adapt your generic frameworks

Once you've learned these generic frameworks, you can start to tailor them to any examination you are taught. For example, here's how you would build the specifics of a cardiovascular examination onto the generic framework of WIPER–IPPA–WaTER, while working anatomically up from the hands (*Table 2.14*). To my mind, it's **much** easier to learn clinical skills this way right from the beginning, rather than reinventing the wheel each time you're taught a new examination.

**Table 2.14: Example of how to adapt your generic examination frameworks to the specifics of a cardiovascular examination.** Note that not all parts of IPPA are required at every stage: there is no percussion in a cardiovascular exam, for example. This is what I mean by adapting the framework to the specific examination.

| Generic framework | Specific to cardiovascular examination |
|---|---|
| WIPER | • Wash your hands<br>• Introduce yourself and get informed consent to examine their heart and circulatory system<br>• Ask the patient if they are in pain<br>• Expose them from the waist up<br>• Position them at 45° on the bed |
| End of the bed | • INSPECTION: look for ECG monitoring, medicines such as a GTN spray and observe the patient's general status |
| Hands | • INSPECTION: look for tar staining, clubbing, splinter haemorrhages, Osler nodes and Janeway lesions<br>• PALPATION: feel if their hands are sweaty, check capillary refill time, pulse and radial-radial delay |
| Arms | • AUSCULTATION: manually check blood pressure (in an OSCE, you can usually just offer to do this) |
| Face | • INSPECTION: look for xanthelasma, corneal arcus, conjunctival pallor, malar flush, central cyanosis and dental hygiene |
| Neck | • INSPECTION: check JVP<br>• PALPATION: feel carotid pulse |
| Chest/back | • INSPECTION: look for scars and a pacemaker/ICD<br>• PALPATION: feel for heaves and thrills<br>• AUSCULTATION: listen to heart sounds, with and without cardiac manoeuvres, and to posterior lung bases |
| Legs | • INSPECTION: look for ankle oedema and vein harvesting scars<br>• PALPATION: feel for ankle oedema |
| WaTER | • Wash your hands<br>• Thank the patient<br>• Cover them up and make sure they are comfortable<br>• Report your findings |

## 2.7.4 Practise, practise, practise

I've watched hundreds of medical students perform examinations and take histories, and there is always one immediate question that pops into my head: do they actually know what they're doing? And it's usually very easy to answer, as it becomes clear within seconds whether they have practised this particular skill before or are just bumbling their way through it. Believe me, it's blindingly obvious!

The reason it's so obvious is because of muscle memory. When you practise a skill hundreds of times, it becomes completely instinctive: your hands and body will start to move on autopilot, following the same patterns they have followed all those countless times before. You become smoother, quicker and more polished, and the whole process gets easier and requires less effort. You simply can't fake muscle memory, which is why it's so easy for an outside observer to recognise whether or not you've truly got it. The same is true for history taking: the more you practise, the more instinctively you will flow from section to section without awkwardly pausing to remember whether it's the drug history or social history that comes next.

> Find a group of friends to start practising clinical and communication skills with as early as possible. This will help you build up muscle memory to get slick, quick and competent.

**TOP TIP**

For this reason, there are no hacks, shortcuts or workarounds for clinical and communication skills. Sorry! You simply have to practise, practise, practise – then go away and practise some more. Every time you are taught a new skill, you should aim to practise it within the next week while it is still fresh in your mind, then keep doing so regularly until it becomes completely instinctive. Set up a weekly study group to run through all the skills you have learned, then go home and practise on your housemates, your partner, your friends, your teddies and yourself. I subjected my wife and children to plenty of clinical skills practice (fortunately my kids find it hilarious to be percussed) and spent some serious time locating every pulse in my body. Just do whatever works for you!

There are two main benefits to all this practice:

1. Get slick: the more ingrained the muscle memory, the slicker and more professional you will look and feel. This will help you develop quicker as a doctor and get you a lot more marks in OSCEs.

2. Free up brainpower: if you have to devote it all to thinking about which step comes next, you have less available for thinking about your

findings and formulating a differential diagnosis. You will therefore start to miss important things and be less prepared to present your findings at the end. By contrast, if your history or examination is flowing freely on autopilot, you can devote all that lovely brainpower to looking, listening, feeling and thinking about what the patient is showing and telling you.

## 2.7.5  Stick to the script

At this early stage of medical school, you will probably be taught to do everything in a very rigid, particular way when it comes to clinical and communication skills, but (**SPOILER ALERT**) fast forward a few years and you will realise that there is an absolutely massive amount of variation in practice. Once you hit the wards, you'll quickly notice that every doctor does things differently, and some might even encourage you to freestyle or tell you that what you were taught is wrong and you should do it their way instead.

This is all well and good later in your training, when you can tinker with your technique to your heart's content (in fact it's absolutely essential that you **do** evolve and develop these skills, and we will look at exactly how to do that in later chapters of this book). But during the preclinical years, I would advise you to strongly resist this temptation, and instead stick religiously to the script that your medical school has taught you. Follow the steps exactly as you were taught, using the techniques you were shown, and don't customise, deviate or try anything fancy.

> **TOP TIP**
>
> During preclinical years, practise clinical skills exactly as taught by your medical school. You will learn to customise them in later years, but don't get ahead of yourself yet.

Why? Because this is the standard against which you will be marked in your OSCEs. And right now, I'm afraid to say, this is the most immediate and pressing priority for you.

**OSCE examiners have a rigid, inflexible mark scheme, and will have just watched 20 other students perform the exact same examination one after the other. If you come in and do something different, they're not going to applaud your creativity and free-spirited individualism – they'll just assume you're a piss-taker who wasn't paying attention in class.**

In the real world, there is huge variation in how doctors take histories and perform clinical examinations. But for your OSCEs, you'll be expected to do it exactly as you were taught!

**KEY POINT**

Later on, when you are free from the shackles of OSCEs, you can shift your priorities towards developing your own style, adding versatility, flair and panache. But until then, your goal is simply to do the exact same thing as everyone else, but **better**.

In fact this issue will rear its head long before you hit the wards: as soon as you start looking at clinical skills textbooks, videos and websites you will find there is conflict with what you have been taught. Should I routinely assess for hepatojugular reflux? Should I use Apley's test or McMurray's test for meniscal damage? Should I test sensation with the patient's eyes open or closed? I cannot answer these questions for you: in these situations, you need to just default back to whatever your medical school taught you and treat it as gospel. Essentially, if it's in your clinical skills handbook, it's correct, and if it ain't, it ain't!

If it helps, you can think of it like learning to drive. During lessons, you are taught to feed the wheel between your hands, look over both shoulders before moving off, and to check your rear-view and side mirror before signalling. Now, we all know perfectly well that most people don't do these things in the real world, but you just need to do them in order to pass and then you are free to do what you like (so long as it's safe). It's the same with clinical skills: you might never see a doctor assess for collapsing pulse, test the gag reflex or auscultate for renal bruits in the real world – but you still need to do them while you are learning. Once you have passed finals – the equivalent of the driving test – you are free to relax and drop the unrealistic extra steps, only doing them if you feel that they are relevant and clinically indicated.

## 2.7.6 **Be the guinea pig**

During the early years of clinical and communication skills, a great way to learn is to volunteer to take part in demonstrations as much as possible. Any time the tutor asks for a volunteer, either to examine or be examined, make an effort to step forward, no matter how embarrassing it may seem to have your classmates watch you.

Doing examinations in front of a small audience can be nerve-racking, but you'll remember the experience *far* better than if you were just watching. You'll also get personalised feedback from the tutor, which is invaluable, as you can use it to hone your technique the next time

**TOP TIP**

Volunteer to examine or be examined as much as possible during clinical and communication skills teaching. You will learn a *lot* more than by passively observing.

you practise that skill. And remember that this is a safe space with low expectations – unlike the pressure of an OSCE – so it's a great opportunity to get used to carrying out examinations with other people watching.

Being examined by someone else is also super-informative, because being on the receiving end gives you first-hand experience of how the examination is supposed to feel, and what works and what doesn't. For example, while assessing visual fields, it takes your friend several minutes to figure out where your blind spot is. But once she finds it, and you experience the odd sensation of the coloured dot disappearing, you'll have a much better idea how to do it once it's your turn to examine. So don't hang back: step up and you'll find your skills improve significantly quicker.

### 2.7.7 Summary

In this section, we have looked at the first phase of developing your clinical and communication skills in preparation for clinical placements and OSCEs. The key points are:

- Clinical and communication skills are fun, interactive and a huge step towards becoming a doctor.
- Rely heavily on structured frameworks and mnemonics such as WIPER-IPPA-WaTER to help yourself remember all the steps and keep track of your place.
- Follow the conventional anatomical order that all doctors use, particularly for cardiovascular, respiratory and abdominal examinations.
- Once you have learned these generic frameworks you can adapt them to any examination by building the specific steps on top.
- Practice is absolutely essential for building up your muscle memory and getting fluent at history taking and examination – try to practise at least once a week with your friends.
- During preclinical years, stick to what you were taught and don't customise your examinations yet.
- Volunteer to examine and be examined in front of the group, as this will really help you to learn.

# 2.8 OSCEs: level I

OSCE. Such a small and unassuming word; such a source of utter terror to medical students the world over. Even now, with med school safely behind me, just hearing the word accelerates my bowels to a pace where I'm reaching for the loperamide. OSCEs are the stuff of nightmares – yet they are an essential and unavoidable part of medical school which you will need to get on top of if you are going to survive.

OSCE, as you may already know, stands for Objective Structured Clinical Examination. They're the practical exams by which medical schools assess your clinical, communication and procedural skills. OSCEs are typically a series of timed stations, in which you step into a cubicle and have around 10 or 15 minutes to complete a specific task such as taking a history from a patient or examining a joint or body system. It might be an actor with a made-up story, a real patient with actual signs and symptoms, or just a rubber arm for you to take fake blood from.

> OSCE = Objective Structured Clinical Examination. They bring as much joy to medical students as Christmas does to turkeys.

**KEY POINT**

We will talk a lot about OSCEs throughout this book, and I will try to demystify the process as much as possible and teach you the essential skills you need to survive. The first steps are to understand the basics: what *are* OSCEs, how do they work and what are the examiners looking for?

## 2.8.1 What to expect

You'll get randomly assigned days and times for your OSCEs, either all in one go or spread out over separate sessions. You show up to a room where everyone waits nervously like lambs before the slaughter, making awkward small talk, fiddling with their stethoscopes, drinking too much water to combat dry mouth then going out to pee an average of 13 times. Eventually, when it's time, they'll line you up in rows and lead you to another room where all the stations are set up – in their own clinical cubicles or behind dividing partitions. You'll be deposited outside your starting station, followed by more excruciating waiting time. Then a buzzer will sound and you'll usually have one minute to read a pre-printed set of instructions outside your station. Then the buzzer sounds again, you step into the station and begin the task assigned to you. There's usually another buzzer towards the end, telling you that you have one minute remaining before moving onto the next station.

**Box 2.17**

**Example tasks in preclinical-year OSCE stations.**
**These typically last 10 or 15 minutes.**

- Take a clinical history from an actor pretending to be a patient and try to work out the diagnosis.
- Explain a procedure or medication to an actor pretending to be a patient.
- Examine someone's knee, shoulder, abdomen or any other body system and present your findings.
- Interpret some basic test results.
- Perform a procedure such as taking blood or inserting a cannula, usually on a rubber arm.

Stations can vary in their structure: sometimes you just run straight through the task however you see fit; in others the examiner will stop you to ask questions, give you some results to interpret or inform you of a new development with the patient. This should be explained in the instructions, so that you can brace yourself for what is coming.

The complexity of stations tends to increase as you get further into medical school – at this early stage of med school, they are typically quite 'clean' and straightforward: you will usually have just a single task to do, with no twists or hidden tricks. My first-year stations, for example, were 10 minutes each and almost all involved actors or healthy volunteers with no clinical findings. Tasks included a respiratory examination, some straightforward medical histories and simple procedures like measuring blood pressure and doing a urine dip.

In the preclinical years, you are **not** expected to know everything or to be the finished product, so don't drive yourself mad by setting unrealistic standards for yourself.

> **Early OSCEs are mainly about ensuring that you are polite, respectful, professional and competent enough to proceed to the clinical years and be let loose on real patients. In other words: practise, stick to what you were taught, don't be an arsehole, and you will be absolutely fine!**

## 2.8.2  How to prepare

Consciously or not, your OSCE preparations are already well underway from learning clinical and communication skills, as discussed in **Section 2.7**.

However, there are some specific things you should do as OSCEs approach, to ensure you build on all that lovely practice you've done so far. Here are ten suggestions:

1.  Practise in threes, where the third student is an observer/examiner. Give each other constructive feedback and take it on board.

2.  Don't neglect history taking and communication skills: these are guaranteed to come up in some form or another, so practise as much as possible using role plays and scenarios from textbooks and websites. A standard clinical history should be second nature to you by OSCE time, and you should be able to adapt it to common high-yield presentations like headache, shortness of breath or chest pain.

3.  Practise under timed conditions, allowing a minute or two at the end for summarising and presenting your findings. Start to think more carefully about your pacing; for example, am I spending too long on my introduction? Why do I always get bogged down in the history of the presenting complaint and never get around to family and social history?

4.  Mimic the OSCE setting by practising in your clinical skills suite or spare clinical cubicles. This will get you used to the amount of space you have to work in and practicalities such as positioning the patient properly on a hospital bed and examining from their right-hand side.

5.  Attend any revision sessions offered by the medical school. No matter how confident you feel, there is always room to improve.

6.  Gradually increase the frequency of your practice sessions as OSCE day approaches. Like training for a marathon, the key is to reach peak performance on the day itself: don't tire yourself out too early, or leave everything too late.

7.  Speak to students in the years above to get a feel for the general flavour of OSCEs at your medical school and which stations tend to come up. This information is invaluable!

8.  Mock OSCEs are an absolute essential. Some student societies run these, or you can get a group of mates together and do it yourselves. Take it seriously: replicate the number of stations and timings that you will face on the day, use proper mark schemes and make sure everyone gets useful feedback. This will get you accustomed to the time pressure and rapid changeovers between stations, making you **much** more prepared for the real thing. I cannot stress highly enough how useful mock OSCEs are – **do them**!

9. Video yourself during practice sessions and watch it back afterwards. This will feel weird and uncomfortable but you can learn absolutely loads about yourself that you might not otherwise have realised, particularly your body language and mannerisms.

10. Brainstorm with friends about what sort of questions an examiner might ask you towards the end of a station. Start building these into your practice sessions so you get used to thinking on your feet.

### 2.8.3 Getting in the zone

I always found it helpful to think of OSCEs as an audition. You are an actor auditioning for the role of doctor in a TV show, and the examiner is the director deciding whether or not you've got what it takes to play the part. In other words, you need to deliver a **performance** in which you convince the examiner that you would make a good doctor. So you will need to inhabit your role by dressing, behaving, speaking and thinking like a doctor. It doesn't matter how nervous and very-very-far-from-being-a-doctor you feel on the inside – you just need to put on a decent show on the outside.

This mindset helped me to deal with nerves, which are a real killer in OSCEs. There'll be lots of well-meaning people who tell you: 'just relax and don't be nervous', but personally that just made me even more nervous! It's not easy to just switch it off like that. So instead I tell myself: "Yes, you're nervous, and that is completely natural and understandable. Accept this fact, then throw yourself into **acting** like you're not nervous. Force yourself to stride purposefully into the station, stand up straight, shake the patient's hand, make eye contact, speak clearly and **pretend** to be confident. Then follow the steps one after another, exactly as you learned them, and keep on moving forwards."

**TOP TIP**

> Accept that you will be nervous in OSCEs. Just *pretend* not to be, and if you do a good enough job of pretending then the examiner won't know the difference.

Before you know it you will find you are flying through the station and the examiner is none the wiser about how nervous you really are. They aren't mind readers, and they're not monitoring your heart rate, sweat levels or bowel transit speed, as far as I'm aware. So if you look calm and confident on the outside, then ultimately what's the difference if you feel like a wreck on the inside?

## 2.8.4 **Learn what the examiners want**

An absolutely crucial step in understanding OSCEs is to get your head around the marking process. Once you know exactly what examiners are looking for, you can focus on giving it to them.

There is a lot of variation between medical schools, but at their heart OSCEs are fundamentally a tick-box exercise. The examiner has a list of things you are expected to do in that station, and each time you do one of those things you get a tick in that box, securing yourself an extra mark. In a hand and wrist examination, for example, commenting on interosseous muscle wasting will get you a mark, palpating the interphalangeal joints will get you another mark, and assessing grip strength will get you yet another. Crying, begging for mercy or dissing the examiner's mother will all get you zero marks.

To illustrate what I'm talking about, see **Tables 2.15** and **2.16** for example mark schemes for respiratory examination and breathlessness history stations, respectively. Do spend some time looking through these and thinking about how to apply them to your own clinical and communication skills. There are a few particular things I'd like you to note:

- There are tons of marks available for generic steps like your introduction, setup, general inspection and closure. These are easy peasy marks which you should be gaining in every single station. This is why frameworks like WIPER and WaTER are so useful – once you get quick and confident at opening and closing a station, you can whizz through and gobble up these marks.

- You need to deliver both quantity **and** quality: there are lots of different steps to get through in a short space of time, so you do need to work quickly. But just doing a particular thing doesn't necessarily get you full marks for it: you need to do it properly, not just make a rushed half-arsed attempt. This is a difficult balancing act which cuts to the very heart of OSCEs: you need to work fast but not **too** fast, and be thorough but not **too** thorough. Finding that balance is probably the hardest part of OSCEs.

- You are unlikely to get through every step in the time allocated to you. A good strategy is therefore to have an impeccable introduction, general manner and closure, then just do your best with the main parts of the examination and make peace with the fact that you won't manage everything. This approach will get you more marks than obsessing over every specific point in the middle at the expense of the generic points available at the beginning and the end.

**Table 2.15: Example mark scheme for a respiratory system examination**

**Instructions:** Mr Orijit Dhar is a 64-year-old gentleman. Examine his respiratory system.
Time allowed: 6 minutes.

| | | | |
|---|---|---|---|
| 1.  Introduction and orientation | 0 | 1 | 2 |
| 2.  Positions and exposes patient | 0 | 1 | 2 |
| 3.  Ensures patient's comfort | 0 | 1 | 2 |
| 4.  Inspects patient's general appearance | 0 | 1 | 2 |
| 5.  Looks into sputum pot | 0 | 1 | 2 |
| 6.  Inspects and examines hands | 0 | 1 | 2 |
| 7.  Determines rate, rhythm, and character of radial pulse | 0 | 1 | 2 |
| 8.  Tests for asterixis | 0 | 1 | 2 |
| 9.  Inspects head for signs of anaemia and central cyanosis | 0 | 1 | 2 |
| 10.  Assesses jugular venous pressure | 0 | 1 | 2 |
| 11.  Palpates cervical, supraclavicular, infraclavicular, and axillary lymph nodes | 0 | 1 | 2 |
| 12.  Palpates for tracheal deviation | 0 | 1 | 2 |
| 13.  Palpates for cardiac apex | 0 | 1 | 2 |
| 14.  Assesses chest expansion | 0 | 1 | 2 |
| 15.  Percusses chest | 0 | 1 | 2 |
| 16.  Auscultates chest | 0 | 1 | 2 |
| 17.  Tests for vocal resonance or tactile fremitus | 0 | 1 | 2 |

Examiner to ask: "Please summarise your findings and offer a differential diagnosis."

| | | | |
|---|---|---|---|
| 18.  Summarises key findings | 0 | 1 | 2 |
| 19.  Offers an appropriate differential diagnosis | 0 | 1 | 2 |

Examiner's global score

0    1    2    3    4

Patient's global score

0    1    2    3    4

Examiner's comments

| |
|---|
|  |

Total marks possible: 46

Reproduced from *Clinical Skills for OSCEs 5e* (online mock mark schemes).

**Table 2.16: Example mark scheme for a breathlessness history**

**Instructions:** Take a history from 58-year-old Mr Arthur Wenzel who presents with breathlessness. Time allowed: 6 minutes.

| | | | |
|---|---|---|---|
| 1. Introduction and orientation | 0 | 1 | 2 |
| 2. Ensures that patient is comfortable | 0 | 1 | 2 |
| 3. Establishes name, age, and occupation | 0 | 1 | 2 |
| 4. For breathlessness, asks about: onset and progression | 0 | 1 | 2 |
| 5. provoking and relieving factors | 0 | 1 | 2 |
| 6. associated symptoms | 0 | 1 | 2 |
| 7. Assesses severity of breathlessness | 0 | 1 | 2 |
| 8. Asks about previous episodes of breathlessness | 0 | 1 | 2 |
| 9. Asks about cigarette smoking | 0 | 1 | 2 |
| 10. Past medical history, key aspects | 0 | 1 | 2 |
| 11. Drug history, key aspects | 0 | 1 | 2 |
| 12. Family history, key aspects | 0 | 1 | 2 |
| 13. Social history, key aspects | 0 | 1 | 2 |

**Examiner to ask:** *"Please summarise your findings and offer a differential diagnosis."*

| | | | |
|---|---|---|---|
| 14. Summarises key findings | 0 | 1 | 2 |
| 15. Offers an appropriate differential diagnosis | 0 | 1 | 2 |

Examiner's global score

0    1    2    3    4

Actor's global score

0    1    2    3    4

Examiner's comments

| |
|---|
| |

Total marks possible: 38

Reproduced from *Clinical Skills for OSCEs 5e* (online mock mark schemes).

Of course these mark schemes are just examples, and your medical school will have its own way of doing things. Some have moved towards 'domain-based marking', where the checklist is broken down into sections such as introduction, information gathering, differential diagnosis, rapport and professionalism. This gives the examiners more flexibility to grade you well in one area but poorly in another, for example. Ultimately this doesn't really matter, as the overall principles remain the same – just make sure you familiarise yourself with your medical school's way of marking OSCEs and what sort of things they are looking for (they should give you a lecture about it). It would be very unwise to approach your OSCEs without ever considering things from the examiner's perspective as well as your own!

## 2.8.5  Top tips for the day

When your first OSCE does eventually roll around, here are my top tips to help you survive the day:

- Scrub up. It's essential for your image as an aspiring doctor that you look and feel the part. If you walk into a station in shabby clothing with a whiff of body odour, you are already facing an uphill struggle to impress your examiner.

- Read your instructions **very** carefully. It's remarkably easy to miss things or get the wrong end of the stick, which can potentially derail your entire station. There's usually a copy of the instructions inside the station – don't hesitate to stop and read them again if you're unsure.

- Maximise first impressions. Force yourself to smile, make eye contact and speak loudly and clearly the moment you walk into a station. Try to look like you're cool, calm and have done this before.

- State your full name and role. Some medical schools will penalise you for not giving both your first name and surname, or not specifying your exact stage of training.

- Offer a chaperone. Make sure you do this in any station involving intimate body parts or substantially undressing the patient. If in doubt, just offer one – you won't lose marks for doing so, but might lose them if you don't.

- Remember your general inspection. This step is **very** commonly missed under pressure, potentially costing a lot of marks. Make a point of standing at the end of the bed for a few seconds to provide some general observations before diving into the specific parts of the examination.

- Be nice to the patients. If they're actors, convince yourself that they are real patients and be friendly, polite and respectful. Mainly because this is a good way to behave in general, but also because they often contribute to your mark so you really don't want to piss them off.

- Don't get ahead of yourself. We all instinctively want to jump ahead to our findings and diagnosis, but you need to resist this urge and keep working through the steps in the right order. Otherwise it's like delivering the punchline before you've finished telling the joke.

- Ask for a time out. If you feel a station is going badly, there is absolutely no harm in asking for a short pause to think and reconsider your approach. I've done this many times. I don't think examiners mark you down for it, and it allows you to run through things in your head and consider what you might have missed.

- Know when to wrap it up. When the buzzer goes to tell you there is one minute remaining, **force** yourself to stop whatever you're doing and move immediately to your summary and closure. That's an entire section of marks you might miss if you don't get around to it.

- Put the last station behind you. No matter how it went, you simply cannot afford to dwell on it when you've got more stations to get through. Draw a line under it and move on, otherwise you risk one bad station becoming two bad stations, then before you know it you're in a downward spiral of doom. In my experience, the station usually went better than you thought at the time. And even if it was a disaster, you can afford to fail a handful of stations and still comfortably pass, so just write it off and keep moving onwards and upwards.

## 2.8.6  The objectivity question

As we know, OSCE stands for Objective Structured Clinical Examination. No one would argue with the SCE part, but the O is much more controversial and gets a lot of students very worked up. I have heard the comment "There's nothing objective about OSCEs" more times than I can count. Let's consider both sides of this argument, then figure out what it means for you.

The justification for OSCEs being described as objective is the fact that every student has to complete the same task and gets graded using the exact same mark scheme. This is intended to create a level playing field and minimise any bias on the part of the examiner. Hence those rigid tick-box mark schemes: these are all about minimising the examiner's subjective opinions of you and forcing them instead to focus on what you actually said and did. In theory, two different students who performed the task in the exact same way should get exactly the same mark.

This is a very noble aim which we should absolutely support and applaud, because the alternative is to give examiners free rein to mark you however they see fit. And we know enough about human behaviour to know that this would be a **bad** idea: however hard they **tried** to be fair, examiners would end up setting a wide range of different tasks for different students, and subconsciously judging them based on their appearance, voice, and any number of other factors. This would be deeply, catastrophically unfair. So in theory, OSCEs are a heroic attempt to introduce objectivity to an otherwise subjective situation.

**KEY POINT**

Objectivity is a noble aim, but impossible to achieve when running clinical exams for hundreds of students.

In reality, however, there is simply no such thing as objectivity in clinical examinations. It is something noble to aspire to, but it can never truly be achieved. I don't mean this in some highfalutin philosophical way – I'm talking about the practicality of running these things for hundreds of students in a short space of time, with all the logistical constraints and human fallibility that entails. See **Table 2.17** for just a handful of reasons why OSCEs aren't truly objective – and believe me, I could go on!

Faced with this imperfect situation, as with so many things in medical school, all you can do is make peace with it and try not to waste unnecessary energy by getting angry and stressed. OSCEs might not be perfect but they're the best we've got, and they will remain a fact of life for the foreseeable future. If you passionately believe they are unfair, and you have a better solution, then I would love to see you get it out there and change the face of medical education forever! But until that day, I'm afraid you're stuck with them, so you might as well focus your energy on doing the absolute best you can.

## 2.8.7 The 20% rule

Throughout your OSCE preparations, something to keep in mind is the inevitable difference between how well you perform in comfortable surroundings with your friends versus the higher-pressure situation on the day. There are so many unpredictable factors – which tasks come up, which actors/patients you get, how nervous you are – that there is no guarantee you will replicate your best performance. You might be Dr House during practice, yet immediately turn into Dr Nick once you enter the station. Your

**Table 2.17: Four reasons why OSCEs can never be truly objective**

| 1. Actors | Their performances introduce huge variability between stations: some inhabit their role like they're in line for an Oscar; others seem totally uninterested. Some seem to hate you from the get-go; others make friends with you and try to feed you clues when the examiner's not looking. |
|---|---|
| 2. Patients | Med schools are at the mercy of whoever they can get for that day, so variability is again inevitable. An abdominal exam on someone with ascites, seven scars, an ileostomy and transplanted kidney is hardly comparable to one on a healthy bloke with moobs and some belly button dandruff. Yet the exact same mark scheme will be used. |
| 3. Examiners | They are only human, and have their own quirks:<br><br>• They use mark schemes differently: some fill it in as you go; others just observe then fill everything in at the end. Either way, they might forget to tick things you did, or they might tick things you didn't do.<br><br>• There is still subjectivity: if they like the cut of your jib, they'll give you the benefit of the doubt on global score or softer boxes like 'ensures patient's comfort'. And if they don't like you, they won't.<br><br>• Some are just instinctively harsher than others, no matter how much they are told to stick to the checklist.<br><br>• You might know them: your heart sinks when you enter a station and see a notoriously strict professor, or soars when it's your favourite soft-touch PBL tutor. This affects nerves and performance.<br><br>• They are randomly assigned to stations: a consultant psychiatrist examining the psychiatry station will inevitably have more knowledge and higher standards than an orthopaedic surgeon examining the psychiatry station, for example.<br><br>• It's a *long* day: they might have to sit through 30 or 40 re-runs of the exact same station. Their attention fluctuates, their blood caffeine level dips and sometimes they're just thinking about how badly they need a wee. |
| 4. Students | • Your performance and confidence vary depending where in the schedule you are assigned. I preferred getting them out of the way early; others preferred going last to maximise preparation time.<br><br>• Examiners are inevitably influenced by who went before you: a string of numpties will make you look good by comparison; a run of whizzkids will make *you* look like the numpty.<br><br>• Some students talk so loudly you can't help overhearing the next station in advance.<br><br>• Some students cheat (see *Section 2.8.8*). |

hands become jelly, your feet freeze to the floor and your brain turns to mush (**Figure 2.14**). I have a friend who regularly struggled to pronounce his own name when introducing himself in OSCEs. And it really wasn't complicated.

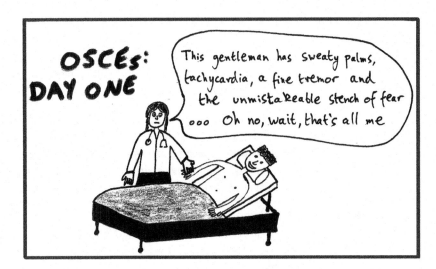

**Figure 2.14: OSCE terror is inevitable and unavoidable.** Brace yourself for it by preparing to the highest standard you can.

As a form of insurance against this problem, I invented something called the 20% rule:

> **However well you perform in practice, you should always assume that you will perform *20% worse* on the day.**

This helps to guard against complacency where students get cocky about OSCEs because they are super-slick when practising with their friends. Absolutely anyone – even the very best and brightest – can be reduced to a gibbering wreck by OSCEs, and it's wise to brace yourself accordingly.

By extension, it follows that you need to perform to a higher standard during practice than you would need to in order to pass the station on the day. If the pass mark is 50%, for example, and you are happily muddling through your practice sessions picking up 60% of the marks, the 20% rule dictates that your performance will drop by 20 percentage points to 40% on the day, causing you to fail that station. If you can bring your practice standard up to 80%, then you can afford to drop down to 60% on the day and still pass. Even better if you're close to 100% during practice, because then you'll pass very comfortably and might even start picking up merits and distinctions. In other words, you need to give yourself a margin of error – a large cushion to fall back onto if OSCE terrors strike.

One personal example of this came during finals when I completely ballsed up a 10-minute cardio-respiratory examination station. I must have practised this skill hundreds of times and felt very comfortable with it. During practice I was confidently nailing the entire exam in seven minutes, eight tops, leaving a couple spare for closure and presenting my findings. There was nothing more I could have done to prepare for this station.

And yet ... I walked in, took one look at the patient and almost immediately lost my mojo. She had nasal cannulae delivering oxygen, connected to a small, fancy-looking device I had never seen before in my life. She also had a huge diagonal scar down one side of her posterior ribcage – clearly something respiratory – but not something I recognised. I nevertheless regained just enough composure to deliver a strong introduction and whizz through the easy bits of the exam, before getting completely thrown off course by the mystery machine and scar. My brain reached desperately for the word for lung removal surgery but drew a blank, leaving me floundering as I attempted to describe my findings. I lost my rhythm, slowed down, and spectacularly failed to complete all the steps of the examination that had been such a doddle in practice. As the buzzer went, telling me I had one minute left, I abandoned ship with the examination unfinished, thanked the patient, covered her up, washed my hands and summarised as best I could.

I came out feeling the station had been a disaster and an absolutely certain fail. So imagine my surprise when I got my marks and discovered I had passed that station. But only by a whisker: I scored 50.0% and the pass mark was 49.8%. I passed by 0.2%. It doesn't get much closer that that!

Why did I pass? Clearly not because of my examination technique or recognition of clinical signs, both of which absolutely sucked on the day, but because everything else I did was good enough to drag my overall score up *just* enough to scrape through. A strong introduction, confident whip-through the easy bits of the exam, some solid rapport and professionalism, and a decent attempt at closure. This is OSCE strategy in a nutshell: pick up as many easy marks as you can to give yourself margin for error if the sh*t hits the fan. Hopefully this won't happen often: in the majority of stations everything will go well and you'll score very highly. Just use the 20% rule to prepare yourself that things won't *always* go exactly according to plan!

(In case you are wondering, with retrospect I figured out it was a *pneumonectomy* scar – of course the word came back to me as soon as I left the station – and a device for delivering humidified home oxygen, just a much snazzier one than those I had seen previously.)

Guard against the 20% rule by practising to the highest standard you can. This will give you room for error on the day.

**TOP TIP**

## 2.8.8  To cheat or not to cheat

To complete our discussion of OSCEs, we must also dip into a taboo subject people do not like to talk openly about: cheating. There is a good chance you will be offered the opportunity to cheat during medical school OSCEs – plenty of your peers will be at it – and I think you would be wise to consider your position and make an informed decision in advance.

What do I mean by cheating? Let's leave aside high-level, proper devious stuff and focus instead on the much more widespread practice of sharing OSCE stations in advance. This is when people from the first group to participate in the OSCE each day message their friends afterwards, telling them which stations are included. They will then tell **their** friends, who tell **their** friends, and so on.

I have absolutely no idea how common this practice is: there is not a lot of research on it, but one estimate suggests around 25–35% of medical students admit to cheating when surveyed anonymously.[4] My personal impression, for what it's worth, is that those figures are an underestimate – the sharing of OSCE stations felt widespread and normalised, to the point where I sometimes felt like a weirdo for not joining in. I received direct offers to trade information, and knew of students who would brazenly phone around people from the morning sessions to try to extract information from them. It got to the point where when heading into medical school for an OSCE, and bumping into people who had already finished their session, I would immediately ask them not to tell me anything, because they seemed like they would automatically spill the beans otherwise.

Personally, I refused to take part because I just think it's wrong to cheat. It saddens me that I should even need to spell that out, but there you go. And reassuringly, I did know lots of other students who felt the same way, and were just as frustrated by this as I was. But by and large, it's clear the moral/ethical angle alone does not carry much weight, so I won't bang on about it.

Instead, I will offer a more pragmatic reason why you shouldn't cheat: I genuinely, hand on heart, 100% believe that it is **not** in your best interests to do so. Or, to put it the other way around, I think you will perform considerably better in OSCEs if you **don't** know what the stations are in advance. This probably seems counterintuitive but hear me out, and hopefully I can persuade you around to my point of view.

---

4 *BMJ*, 2015;351:h4014

> Don't cheat in OSCEs. I know they are unpleasant and stressful but I passionately believe that cheating will actually hinder your performance!

**TOP TIP**

Here are nine reasons why knowing the stations in advance is **not** a good idea:

1.  It messes up your structures and thinking patterns. If you already know the diagnosis, you will inevitably tailor your history and examination towards it instead of going through all the steps carefully and systematically. You'll miss things, cut corners and overlook important differential diagnoses which – even though you know they're not correct – will still score you extra marks for exploring them properly. Consider a shortness of breath history: you might know it's COPD, but did you **properly** exclude a pulmonary embolism? Heart failure? Anaemia? That's a lot of marks you potentially just dropped.

2.  Complacency creeps in. Yes, OSCEs are scary, but that fear serves a helpful function by keeping you on your toes and forcing you to think quickly and carefully. Without that adrenaline surge, it is easy to get careless and sloppy.

3.  You move slower. Personally, my desire to uncover the diagnosis is what drove me through OSCE stations at speed, because I knew I couldn't relax until I had figured it out. And that proved to be a **good thing** because by moving quicker, you ask more questions, tick more boxes and get more marks in the time available. If you already know the answer, by contrast, that impetus is gone, causing you to work slower and pick up fewer marks.

4.  It totally misses the point of how OSCEs work. There are only a certain number of marks available for getting the diagnosis, so even if you know **exactly** what's coming, you still need to complete all the steps properly to get the marks in the other domains. You'll score higher for doing the perfect history and examination but getting the diagnosis wrong than you will for a sloppy history and examination with the correct diagnosis.

5.  You'll start to second-guess yourself. With that extra knowledge comes a desire to conceal it from the examiner, which can cause you to start overthinking things and twisting yourself in mental knots. "Damn, did that question make it too obvious? Maybe I'd better ask a couple of dumb ones now to throw them off the scent. But what if

my dumb question is **too** dumb, which makes it **even more** obvious?" And so on. That's a lot of added stress and unnecessary brainpower.

**6.** Your conscience might nag at you. Unless you have true sociopathic tendencies, it would be natural to feel a little pang of guilt about walking into a station knowing exactly what to expect. This can gnaw away at you and distract you from the task in hand.

**7.** The information might be wrong. Medical schools do have safeguards in place, such as mixing up the stations and diagnoses within a session. You're going to look pretty silly when you confidently label that acute abdomen as an ectopic pregnancy, only for the examiner to point out that the patient is in fact a man.

**8.** There is potential for serious consequences. If you slip up and get caught, you will almost certainly fail the exam and might face further disciplinary action. The University of Glasgow made all 270 students resit their finals in 2017 after discovering that information about OSCE stations had been shared around, and even referred some to the GMC for fitness to practise hearings. Is it **really** worth that risk for a few extra marks?

**9.** You're undermining your future skills. Sure, the focus **right now** is on OSCEs, but those processes of history taking, examination and diagnostic reasoning will remain fundamental to being a good doctor long after OSCEs are behind you. In the real world, you won't be able to WhatsApp your mate to ask what's wrong with the guy in cubicle 4. You'll need to be able to figure it out for yourself, and OSCEs are where that process begins.

If these arguments don't persuade you, it is worth considering one last, simple question: do you think medical schools don't know that this is going on? Because believe me, on some level they know **very well** that students are swapping information about OSCE stations and yet they allow it to continue. Why? Because they analyse the data, comparing performance between morning sessions and afternoon sessions, between different days, and between different groups of students. And they always conclude the same thing: that if people are indeed cheating, they are not deriving any clear benefit in terms of their marks, so there is no real imperative to crack down on it.

**This begs the question: why on earth would you risk everything you have worked for when there is no clear evidence you will even benefit?**

It's a huge risk for a small reward, and the negative consequences are potentially life-changing. But hey, it's a free country, so you do whatever you think is best!

## 2.8.9 Summary

In this section, we have taken our first look at OSCEs, including what to expect and how to prepare. The key points are:

- OSCEs can be stressful and unpleasant but unfortunately you will have to get used to them.
- Stations are usually straightforward at this stage and expectations not too high: they basically want to see that you appear competent, polite and professional.
- In the run-up to OSCEs, build on your existing clinical and communication skills by practising under timed conditions with a friend observing and providing feedback.
- Do mock OSCEs: they're absolutely brilliant practice.
- Nerves are inevitable. Just do your best to fool the examiner into thinking you're calm and confident.
- Spend some time going over mark schemes to understand what examiners are looking for.
- On the day, dress smartly, read instructions carefully, be nice to actors and patients and make sure to wrap stations up when the penultimate buzzer goes.
- Don't dwell on the previous station as this can really drag you down.
- OSCEs aren't objective. Get over it.
- Expect to perform at least 20% worse on the day than during practice.
- Lots of people will cheat. It's not in your best interests to be one of them.

# 2.9 Written exams

Written exams are absolutely no one's idea of fun. For me, revision period meant stockpiling junk food, reducing showering from OD to PRN then withdrawing from my already pathetic social life to disappear under mountains of notes for days at a time. I'd have worn DVT socks, if it hadn't meant leaving the house to buy them. And then there's the day itself: a wobbly desk in a freezing cold sports hall, other students casually mentioning topics you've literally never heard of and the inevitable last-minute panic about whether your pencil is HB. Give me a bollocking from a scary consultant any day.

Still, you're stuck with exams, so we need to think about how you can best prepare yourself for them. Like with so much of medical school, exams are all about proper preparation: it's unwise to simply charge into your exam period without a sensible plan. So as soon as you are approaching revision time I'd suggest you sit yourself down to make a seriously good revision timetable. You can devote several hours to this job – it is time excellently spent!

## 2.9.1 Making a revision timetable

A good revision timetable is all about managing the 3Ts: time, topics and techniques, as shown in **Table 2.18**. Ensure you spread your time evenly between the topics and select the right techniques to make the information stick. It's very important during this planning phase to take a bird's eye view across the whole curriculum to ensure you aren't missing any big subjects. **Table 2.19** provides an example based on one of my old revision timetables. Of course revision timetables are a very personal thing – not everything that worked for me will work for you – but hopefully this will at least help illustrate some of the key principles.

**TOP TIP**

When devising a revision timetable, make sure the topics you intend to cover are clearly defined and realistically achievable in the time allocated.

One final piece of advice about revision period: there is a strong tendency among med students to skive off timetabled activities as soon as exams appear on the horizon, in order to get revision done. This is understandable and makes sense up to a point – but be careful not to take it to the extreme of falling behind in your teaching programme, as this can be totally counterproductive. You'll just have to catch up later on the stuff you've missed, so you've not saved yourself much time in the long run. Try

**Table 2.18: Planning for exam period.** There are three main things to consider when making a revision timetable: how to allocate your time, which topics you intend to cover and which techniques you plan to use.

| Time | Topics | Techniques |
|---|---|---|
| • Start in plenty of time before your exams; I usually made my timetable at least 6 weeks in advance<br><br>• Work out how much time you have left between now and exams and when you are free to study<br><br>• Break your time down into one-week blocks, which you can assign revision subjects to<br><br>• Allocate more time to areas where you feel weak than those where you feel strong<br><br>• At the end of each week allow at least half a day for consolidating everything you have covered that week, for example by self-testing, making flashcards, doing MCQs or re-reading and editing your notes | • Make a list of all the major subjects you intend to cover (e.g. cardio, gastro) and divide up the weeks between them; aim for two or three per week – it's better to be ambitious than make a timetable that doesn't stretch you<br><br>• Within each major subject, keeping rolling lists of all the specific, smaller topics you still need to cover (for example 'the cardiac cycle' would be a specific topic within cardiology)<br><br>• Try to match revision topics to things you are already covering that week during your timetabled hours in lectures, tutorials or placements<br><br>• Define your revision topics clearly and make sure they are realistic and achievable in the time frame<br><br>• Cover high-yield topics first and in more detail, and leave the smaller-print stuff till later<br><br>• At the end of each week, update your list to reflect which topics you did and didn't cover, then *move on*; don't stress about not getting around to everything, otherwise you'll get bogged down and fall behind | • Mix up your techniques and resources, matching them to the topics you are studying, e.g. drawings for anatomy, flashcards for physiology, mind maps for pathology<br><br>• Keep testing yourself to prove the knowledge is sticking<br><br>• Lock in some group study sessions with your friends, particularly for OSCE practice (Wednesday afternoons are a great regular spot if you're not in sports teams)<br><br>• Find out if your med school is offering revision lectures and try to go along or watch them online<br><br>• Factor in time for yourself to exercise, go for walks and socialise/leave the house *just* enough to keep yourself sane (I had strict rules of never studying on Friday or Saturday nights, and ensuring I exercised at least twice a week, but find whatever works for you) |

**Table 2.19: Example of a week's revision timetable from my first year.** I've assigned two additional revision subjects to the week, on top of the main subject being taught during that week's scheduled teaching (haematology, in this case). Within each major subject, I've picked a few key topics to cover along with some resources and techniques which I had used previously. This list of revision topics is small but each topic is clearly defined, high-yield and achievable in the time frame.

| Extra revision subjects | Monday | Tuesday | Wednesday | Thursday | Friday | Saturday | Sunday |
|---|---|---|---|---|---|---|---|
| | TEACHING: HAEMATOLOGY | TEACHING: HAEMATOLOGY | TEACHING: HAEMATOLOGY | TEACHING: HAEMATOLOGY | TEACHING: HAEMATOLOGY | a.m.: swim then finish remaining haem topics | a.m.: finish remaining rheum topics |
| 1. Endocrinology | a.m.: PBL | a.m.: haem lectures | a.m.: PBL | a.m.: dissection | a.m.: PBL | p.m.: finish remaining endo topics | p.m.: *consolidation* |
| 2. Rheumatology | p.m.: SDL: blitz haem LOBs in the library to get ahead for the week | p.m.: clinical and comm skills. Revise endo in library afterwards. | p.m.: OSCE practice: endocrine and rheum histories, hand and wrist exam | p.m.: haem lectures | p.m.: go over rheum LOBs in study group | | |
| | Evening: revise endo | Evening: endocrine revision lecture | Evening: play football | Evening: revise rheum | EVENING OFF | EVENING OFF | Evening: plan for next week |

**Key topics:**

- Haematology: different types of leukaemia (see Khan Academy vids), myeloma (re-read notes and Dr Deac Pimp), interpretation of FBC and clotting test results (make flashcards based on lecture slides)

- Endo: diagnostic criteria for diabetes (see PassMed summary), thyroid disease (watch Handwritten Tutorials, practise drawing T3/T4 feedback loops from memory), Cushing's disease vs. syndrome (make a table and mind map based on Tortora textbook and lecture slides)

- Rheumatology: revise hand and wrist anatomy (Netter's flashcards) and link this to deformities in rheumatoid and osteoarthritis (lecture slides, clinical skills handbook), gout (see Dr Deac Pimp), pharmacology of NSAIDs (go over this in study group)

*Consolidation* = practise MCQs and flashcards on endocrinology, rheumatology and haematology. Take stock of which topics I did and didn't manage to cover over the course of the week and how well I feel I know them. Update notes and flashcards accordingly.

to find a good balance between learning new material and revising the subjects you have already covered.

## 2.9.2 **How to revise**

Hopefully your revision will flow naturally from your timetable but if you are struggling, I would recommend a quick look back to **Chapter 1** at some of the coping skills we discussed, as these really come into their own during revision period. It can be a very stressful time and it is important to put your health first and foremost – any exam which destroys you in the process is simply not worth taking. Period.

Don't let your revision timetable become a source of stress: if you've inadvertently set yourself overly ambitious targets which you fail to meet, that is absolutely fine! I did it all the time. Just accept that you missed some stuff and keep ploughing on: if you only managed to cover three of the five endocrinology topics you intended to do in a day, for example, don't automatically devote another day to it because you will start to fall behind on other subjects. Just keep a list of stuff you didn't get around to and then you can come back to it nearer the time, even if just for a quick skim. Remember these subjects are infinite and there will **always** be more you could have done, so try to make your peace with that. It is better to cover those three topics properly than to get yourself in a flap trying to do all five and ending up doing a half-arsed job of all of them.

> Some subjects just **will not** stick in your brain, no matter how hard you try (for me the brachial plexus, clotting cascade and vitamin D metabolism were key culprits). If this is the case, just ram them into your short-term memory the day before the exam or even on the morning of. You only need this sort of information to stay there for a few hours – never mind if you can't remember it the day after!

**TOP TIP**

In terms of resources, you should start to increase your use of practice papers, online question banks and MCQ books as exams approach, as well as all the other techniques for self-testing we have discussed. Official practice papers from your medical school are the most valuable resource of all, because they are written in the right style and tend to address topics with a high chance of coming up. You can get more value out of these papers by attempting them as soon as you receive them, then putting them away for long enough that you forget the questions and can attempt them again with a clean slate. Keep track of topics that pop up regularly, and make extra notes and flashcards if you need to boost your knowledge

**TOP TIP**

Gradually ramp up your use of practice papers, online question banks and MCQ books as exams approach. You can easily get bored of these resources if you use them too early, so it's good to keep them fresh for revision periods.

of these areas. Any time you get a question wrong you should try to learn from it so that you can get it right next time – don't just shrug your shoulders and move on!

### 2.9.3  What to do on the day

I don't want to sound like your mother so I'm not going to tell you to get a good night's sleep before an exam, eat a hearty breakfast and arrive in plenty of time. But that is damn sensible advice, so you should probably listen to her. Also make sure you keep hydrated during the exam (but not so hydrated you need to pee three minutes into it), pace yourself and read the questions carefully. Timekeeping is the number one challenge in med school exams, so keep a very close eye on the clock, force yourself to keep moving forwards and don't let individual questions slow you down too much. Answer every question, even if you have to guess a few towards the end.

### 2.9.4  How to read MCQs

You've already aced your A-levels and got into medical school, so by now you are a pro at taking written exams and coping with pressure. There is really just one thing you need to do differently for medical school, which is to change the way you read MCQs.

Essentially, the problem is this: those sneaky people who write the questions have deliberately packed them full of unnecessary, extraneous guff just to slow you down, waste your time and throw you off course. I know, right? This should be illegal. But it's not and they do it all the time, so you need to outsmart them and stay one step ahead.

The way to do that is to learn to **filter** – to develop a reading style which extracts the key information within seconds and leaves all the extra padding behind on the page. The best way to do this is to flick your eyes down to the actual question at the bottom before you read any of the introductory stem. This may seem counter-intuitive because you are skipping to the end before you've read the beginning, but it will save

When approaching multiple-choice exam questions, start by flicking your eyes down to the end to establish what the actual question is before you invest time in reading the introductory stem. Then you can go back and read the stem more efficiently by extracting only the information needed to answer the question, while filtering out all the unnecessary extra waffle.

**TOP TIP**

you an **enormous** amount of time. Because once you know what you are looking for, you can go back to the start and skim through the stem much quicker, just extracting the key information which actually helps you answer the question. Often you'll discover most of the stem is irrelevant! But if you just start reading it straight away, without knowing what you are looking for, you can waste several minutes before realising this.

Here's a real example question to illustrate what I'm talking about:

*An 18-year-old man is brought to see his GP by his parents. They are concerned about his behaviour. It takes him 2 hours to get ready in the morning. He has a very set routine, including cleaning the bathroom, and then washing himself. He explains he has to clean himself in a particular way, and finishes by washing his hands 11 times. The cleaning routine takes him about 2 hours. If he is interrupted he has to start the routine from the very beginning. The skin on his hands is very dry and scaly. He gets very frustrated by his cleaning, and wishes he didn't have to do this. He accepts that he is not dirty or contaminated. If he tries to resist he becomes distressed and describes multiple unpleasant physical symptoms of anxiety. He continues to worry that he is dirty, and washes his hands throughout the day. When he gets home, he has to take off his clothes immediately and put these in the washing machine before showering again. He has tried to make his parents do the same thing in case they are contaminated, but they have so far refused. The GP thinks he has an obsessive–compulsive disorder.*

*Which of the following is most important when making this diagnosis?*

*A. Asking about a family history of obsessive–compulsive disorder.*
*B. Checking that the patient believes the thoughts are his own.*
*C. Checking the core and other symptoms of depression.*
*D. Checking the patient's insight into his presentation.*
*E. The symptoms need to have been present for 1 week.*

Forget the answer for a second – just look how bloody long that question stem is! It's 202 words! If every question was this long, and you read through them all properly, you'd be lucky to get through half the exam before the buzzer went. Now look at the question again in **Figure 2.15**. As you can see, this turns out to be a generic question about how to diagnose OCD, which doesn't actually relate to the patient himself. You can still answer it

> *An 18-year-old man is brought to see his GP by his parents. ~~They are concerned about his behaviour. It takes him 2 hours to get ready in the morning. He has a very set routine, including cleaning the bathroom, and then washing himself. He explains he has to clean himself in a particular way, and finishes by washing his hands 11 times. The cleaning routine takes him about 2 hours. If he is interrupted he has to start the routine from the very beginning. The skin on his hands is very dry and scaly. He gets very frustrated by his cleaning, and wishes he didn't have to do this. He accepts that he is not dirty or contaminated. If he tries to resist he becomes distressed and describes multiple unpleasant physical symptoms of anxiety. He continues to worry that he is dirty, and washes his hands throughout the day. When he gets home, he has to take off his clothes immediately and put these in the washing machine before showering again. He has tried to make his parents do the same thing in case they are contaminated, but they have so far refused.~~ The GP thinks he has an obsessive–compulsive disorder.*
>
> *Which of the following is most important when making this diagnosis?*
>
> *A. Asking about a family history of obsessive–compulsive disorder.*
> *B. Checking that the patient believes the thoughts are his own.*
> *C. Checking the core and other symptoms of depression.*
> *D. Checking the patient's insight into his presentation.*
> *E. The symptoms need to have been present for 1 week.*

**Figure 2.15: Example of a multiple-choice exam question containing a huge amount of waffle in the introductory stem.** It turns out you don't actually need any of the background information to answer the question because you are told that the diagnosis is OCD! It then becomes a generic question about how to confirm this diagnosis. If you can mentally edit like this, you'll save yourself precious minutes in exams which might otherwise have been wasted. The answer is B, by the way, as this distinguishes the diagnosis of OCD from psychosis and schizophrenia.

This question is reproduced from *Psychiatry: a clinical handbook* (Azam et al., 2016), with permission.

just as easily with the entire stem removed. So all of that information about his symptoms, although interesting and important in real life, is totally irrelevant for this MCQ! This might seem like an extreme example but it's actually very common: there are **a lot** of questions like this at medical school, and you can save yourself a serious amount of time in exams by developing this skill over the years.

> Hone your skill at filtering questions in advance, using practice papers and online question banks. Don't be trying it for the first time during real exams or you might come unstuck!

**TOP TIP**

## 2.9.5 Summary

In this section, we have looked at how to approach written exams in preclinical years. The key points are:

- Invest some proper time and effort into making a revision timetable.
- Focus on the 3Ts: time, topics and techniques. Define topics clearly, divide your time up equally between them and choose your techniques carefully.
- Keep showing up to teaching during revision period so you don't fall behind.
- Revision period can be stressful – remember some of the coping skills we learned in **Chapter 1**.
- Build up your use of MCQs and practice papers as exam time approaches.
- Try to learn from any practice question you get wrong.
- Time pressure can be intense in written exams: learn to extract the key information quickly by skipping to the end of questions so you know what you are looking for before you read the stem.

Good luck in your exams and I'll see you in clinical year one!

# Chapter 3
# Your first clinical year

## Contents

# 3.1 What's it all about?

Your first clinical year is a huge milestone in medical school. It's the point where you cease being purely a university student and begin morphing into a doctor in training. At my medical school, St George's, this year was called transition year (or T-year for short) – a name that makes this point very nicely. This transition involves changing the way you study, think, behave and even dress. Your days of rolling out of bed at 8.50 and slinging on some trackie bums for a 9 a.m. lecture are now, tragically, over. May they rest in peace.

For us, T-year alternated between clinical and university-based blocks, which provided a nice gentle introduction to clinical placements. For many students, however, you'll be thrown straight into the deep end of full-time clinical blocks without the university time to cushion your fall. For this reason, this chapter will focus predominantly on clinical placements, especially since you will be encountering these for the first time. We will, however, look briefly at academic study first so that you can continue to maximise your learning throughout the year.

# 3.2 Techniques

By this stage, you've already had between one and three years of preclinical study and will already know which techniques work for you and which don't. Rather than continuing to experiment with new approaches, therefore, I would suggest that you stick to the tried and tested strategies you have already developed, but focus on evolving the content and style. Your goals are to shift the content away from basic science and onto more clinically focused topics, and to shift the style from long study sessions to shorter, more intense bursts of learning, since you will have less time to spare. See **Table 3.1** for an example of this.

**KEY POINT**

In the clinical years, the *content* of your studying should naturally shift from basic science to more clinically focused topics such as understanding signs and symptoms, ordering and interpreting investigations, making diagnoses and initiating management. You are moving away from abstract ideas and concepts and onto the specifics of what you as a doctor would need to do for actual patients.

**Table 3.1: Example of evolving the content and style of your studies for the clinical years.** Here's how a clinical-years student might go about studying the topic of hypertension, as compared to a preclinical student.

| Preclinical years | Clinical years |
|---|---|
| • Understand the physiological relationships between cardiac output, stroke volume and systemic vascular resistance<br><br>• Get your head around the renin–angiotensin–aldosterone system and the mechanism of drugs that act on it<br><br>• Consider the molecular structure of alpha and beta adrenoceptors and their intracellular signalling cascades<br><br>• Pore over histology slides to learn the different layers of blood vessels and how they change with age<br><br>• Look at pathology books for cool pictures of hypertensive hearts and atherosclerotic blood vessels at autopsy<br><br>• Delve into secondary causes of hypertension such as adrenal tumours to figure out the underlying pathophysiology<br><br>• Learn the embryological formation of blood vessels | • Learn how to diagnose hypertension and the criteria for classifying its different stages<br><br>• Understand which investigations are required to exclude secondary causes of hypertension<br><br>• Know the pharmacological management of hypertension inside out, particularly the NICE algorithm dictating which patients should be started on which drugs<br><br>• Focus on indications, side-effects, interactions and monitoring of drugs, rather than mechanisms<br><br>• Know the complications of hypertension and how to monitor for them<br><br>• Have some idea about the population-level burden of hypertension and what sort of screening and risk-reduction strategies are deployed in the UK<br><br>• Realise that knowing the embryology of blood vessels serves no practical purpose whatsoever to junior doctors |

> Try to study in shorter, more intensive bursts than in previous years. This approach is better suited to being on clinical placements where you may not have big chunks of free time for SDL.

TOP TIP

This sort of evolution should apply to whichever study techniques you use and whichever topics you cover. If you enjoy group study, for example, your sessions should be moving away from epic diagrams of synapses and lengthy conversations about neurotransmitters and onto the diagnosis and management of depression and the role of SSRIs. If you're a fan of making your own flashcards, start testing yourself on chest X-ray findings and blood results in pneumonia rather than its epidemiology and pathophysiology. If mnemonics are your thing, start prioritising clinical ones like MONARCH over anatomical ones like SAIL.[1]

---

1 MONARCH is for the management of acute coronary syndromes: Morphine, Oxygen, Nitrates, Aspirin, Relocate to CCU, Clopidogrel, Heparin. SAIL is for the anatomical boundaries of the femoral triangle: Sartorius, Adductor longus, Inguinal Ligament.

You should also start to focus *a lot* more on investigations at this stage of medical school. ECGs, chest and abdominal X-rays, ABGs, routine blood tests and spirometry are a good place to start: these are all extremely high-yield and almost guaranteed to come up in exams. Look at them on placements whenever possible and discuss them with junior doctors. It's also vital to practise interpreting and presenting investigations with your friends, so that you get into the habit of analysing and describing things out loud in a less pressurised environment (see **Section 3.6.6** for more).

**TOP TIP**

Devote some serious time to interpreting the following investigations as they are virtually guaranteed to come up in exams from now on:
- ECGs
- Chest and abdominal X-rays
- Common blood tests: FBC, U&Es, LFTs, TFTs, bone profile, coagulation and CRP
- Arterial blood gases
- Spirometry.

You will probably find that, as your learning style evolves through medical school, you are producing a smaller volume of material but using those materials more often (**Figure 3.1**). Everything becomes

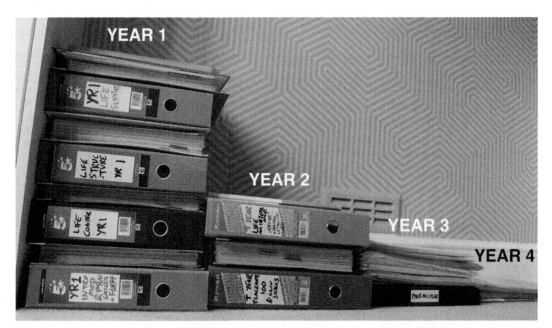

**Figure 3.1: Reducing the volume of material you produce and use throughout medical school.** This photo shows my folders of notes from each of my four years of medical school stacked up alongside each other. Note the year-by-year shrinking in the size of the piles! As I produced fewer notes, I instead became more reliant on single-page summaries, electronic flashcards, online question banks and small, quick-reference textbooks.

more condensed: from reams of notes into short summaries, from lavish drawings into concise tables and mind maps. This is all part of the process of building that skyscraper we talked about in **Section 2.3**: if you can feel this happening then you are well on your way towards the top.

> As you progress through medical school, you will probably use and produce a smaller volume of material but refer more often to the materials you do use. This is an important part of your transition from a student to a junior doctor!

**KEY POINT**

# 3.3 **Resources**

This gradual shift in emphasis from basic science to clinical medicine should also start to manifest in the **type** of resource you use, as well as the quantity. You'll rely less heavily on 'pure' anatomy and physiology sources, for example, and more on sources that integrate these topics with investigations, diagnosis and management. In this section, we'll look at some specific suggestions which are well suited to your first year of clinical placements. We'll also introduce resources for enhancing your clinical, communication and OSCE skills, since you will need to step these up in the clinical years.

Lectures and PowerPoint slides are still useful pointers to what you do and don't need to know (you will probably get a series of lectures at the beginning of each clinical placement); however, do start taking them with a **slight** pinch of salt as their relative importance starts to decline from here on in.

> **If students are being taught across different hospitals, there is no longer any guarantee that the person teaching you is the same person writing your exam questions! So you may need to show a bit more initiative to work out which topics are important and which aren't, rather than trying to second-guess what might come up in exams based on what the lecturer said.**

One way to do this is to consider whether an FY1 would be expected to know a particular piece of information: after all, that's the level of knowledge you're targeting for finals and graduation. If it's something they need to know about, you will need to learn it at some point. If it's too specialist for them, then it's probably too specialist for you too. If you're not sure, just ask an FY1 on your placements!

> Over the years of medical school, try to reduce your reliance on lecture slides to tell you which topics you need to cover. Instead, ask yourself: would an FY1 be expected to know this? If the answer is yes, then you need to know about it too.

### 3.3.1 Books

The first thing to do before the year even starts is buy yourself a small, pocket-sized general medical textbook which you can carry around on placements. If you buy only one book for all of medical school, I'd suggest this is the type to go for because they aren't too expensive, you can potentially get phenomenal use out of it and it creates a better impression than looking stuff up on your phone.

The classic option is the **Oxford Handbook of Clinical Medicine**: known colloquially as The Cheese and Onion, this book is ubiquitous among medical students and junior doctors the world over. Like the old adage about rats in London, I suspect that in a UK teaching hospital you're never more than six feet away from a copy. However, there are so many different options on the market nowadays (see **Table 3.2**), you'd be wise to have a browse in the library or online to see which you like best before committing your cash. You want something accurate, concise and small enough to fit into a handbag or the pocket of scrubs so you can easily whip it out and dig up a quick fact while a consultant is distracted, ready to wow them when their attention returns to you.

> Get yourself a small general medical textbook which can fit into a pocket or handbag. This will come in very handy on clinical placements. Be sure to write your name on it in case someone tries to nick it!

Similarly, you might want to consider a pocket-sized pharmacology book to get you through the clinical years. As we'll see in **Section 3.5**, I'm a huge believer in the importance of learning pharmacology at this stage of medical school: I relied very heavily on **The Top 100 Drugs** (the book that is, not the recreational kind) which is focused on the 'need-to-know' essentials for FY1. But it's not necessarily an essential purchase if you prefer other books or media for pharmacology.

In terms of larger textbooks to study from at home or in the library, you'll find there are absolutely loads of clinically focused options which provide

**Table 3.2: Useful books for your first year of clinical placements**

| Type of book | Why they're helpful | Examples |
|---|---|---|
| Pocket-sized general medical textbook | Small and easy to carry<br><br>Great for quick reference during quiet moments on placement | • *Oxford Handbook of Clinical Medicine*<br>• *Essentials of Kumar and Clark's Clinical Medicine*<br>• *Pocket Medicine*<br>• *Pocket Tutor* series<br>• *Pocket Essentials* series |
| Clinical pharmacology | An essential topic from now until finals; you will need to learn a *huge* amount about drug indications, dosing, side-effects and interactions | • *The Top 100 Drugs*<br>• *Pocket Prescriber*<br>• *Essential Prescribing*<br>• *The Unofficial Guide to Prescribing*<br>• *Prescribing Scenarios At a Glance* |
| Clinically focused textbooks | Useful for bridging the gap between basic sciences and clinical medicine<br><br>Perfect for longer study sessions at home or in the library | • *Kumar and Clark's Clinical Medicine*<br>• *Davidson's Principles and Practice of Medicine*<br>• *Medicine in a Minute*<br>• *First Aid for the USMLE Step 1*<br>• *Data Interpretation for Medical Students*<br>• *The ECG Made Easy* |
| Clinical and communication skills | Help you progress from rote rehearsal to a more realistic style of examination and history taking<br><br>Loads of scenarios for practice and role play | • *Macleod's Clinical Examination*<br>• *OSCE Cases with Mark Schemes: a revision aid for medical finals*<br>• *OSCEs for Medical Finals*<br>• *The Unofficial Guide to Passing OSCEs*<br>• *Essential Examination*<br>• *Clinical Skills for OSCEs*<br>• *The OSCE Revision Guide for Medical Students* |

an excellent bridge between the basic sciences and clinical medicine (***Table 3.2***). These can really help you through this tricky middle phase of medical school when you are still learning how to connect the knowledge from previous years with diagnosis, investigations and management. Also take a look back at ***Table 2.6*** in the previous chapter, as these books are helpful in the clinical years too.

## 3.3.2 Websites

As well as all the websites we mentioned in the last chapter (**Section 2.5.9**), there are a few more which can really help you out in the clinical years:

**Box 3.1**

**Top websites to use in the clinical years**

- *Radiopaedia* (radiopaedia.org) and *Radiology Masterclass* (radiologymasterclass.co.uk). Absolutely essential for improving your interpretation of X-rays. They have tons of great images and quizzes for testing yourself, all available for free.
- *Twitter*: There are loads of great medical accounts and hashtags to follow, such as #FOAMed (free open-access medical education), #MedEd, #SoMeDocs (social media doctors) and #TipsforNewDocs. Lots of specialties have their own too: #CardioTwitter, #PaedsRocks, #NephMadness and #Surgery, to name but a few!
- Clinical Knowledge Summaries from NICE, the National Institute for Health and Care Excellence (cks.nice.org.uk). These are generally more concise and digestible than the full guidelines which accompany them!
- *DermNet* (dermnetnz.org) for all things skin: has an amazing library of images. The British Association of Dermatology website (bad.org.uk/healthcare-professionals/education/medical-students) also has a freely downloadable handbook for medical students which covers everything you need to know to finals level.
- *Life in the Fast Lane* (litfl.com). A blog focusing on emergency medicine. Loads of ECGs, including practice questions.
- *BMJ Learning* (learning.bmj.com). Online educational modules covering a wide range of topics. Free access through your student BMA membership.
- Acadoodle (acadoodle.com): subscription-based online tutorials focusing on ECGs and ABGs.
- *OSCE Pass* (oscepass.com), *OSCE Stop* (oscestop.com) and *MediStudents* (medistudents.com). Free guides to examination and history taking.
- *Scott's Notes* (scottsnotes.co.uk). Free, comprehensive revision guides to medicine, surgery and clinical examination written by Alasdair Scott, who graduated from Imperial in 2012 and is now a surgical registrar.

## 3.3.3 Apps

We mentioned the **BNF, BMJ Best Practice** and **UpToDate** in **Chapter 2**: these are brilliant for clinical placements as they are easy to search and navigate, are regularly updated, can be used offline, and pack an absolutely enormous amount of information into a single place. Also check out:

- **MicroGuide:** this is the major portal for antibiotic guidelines, where you can download specific guidelines for your local trust. **Spectrum: Antimicrobials** is also excellent for general information on antibiotics and pathogens, but specific guidance is currently limited to US hospitals.

- There may also be equivalent apps for other kinds of local guidelines, for example **GreyMobile** provided access to the St George's 'Grey Book' guidelines on the management of common medical emergencies (the app is no longer being updated but is still a useful source of background information). If you're not sure, just ask the FY1s which apps they use.

- **Induction:** this is basically a phone book of all the extensions and bleep numbers in UK hospitals. Perfect for when one of the doctors asks you to call another department or chase up a test result.

- **MDCalc:** a database of commonly used medical calculators and scoring systems. In short, if you can't be bothered to commit the $CHA_2DS_2$-VASc and HASBLED scores to memory (and frankly I don't blame you), then this app is for you.

- **PocketDr:** a handy guide to common situations faced by on-call doctors, including prescribing and the management of acutely unwell patients. You'll have to pay for this one (the others listed here are free).

## 3.3.4 Question banks

We mentioned the big three online question banks in **Chapter 2**: PassMedicine, PasTest and OnExamination. I used these **a lot** during my clinical years, particularly in the run-up to exams. Whichever one you're using, make sure it knows you have moved onto clinical placements and isn't still serving you basic science questions! You have to pay to subscribe to these sites but most students decide they're worth the money and will sign up to at least one each year. They contain extraordinary amounts of information and, in my opinion, have become an essential resource for the modern medical student.

You should try to be smart in how you use these sites, rather than just aimlessly ploughing through huge quantities of questions. Here's how you can get the most out of them:

- Focus on one subject at a time. You can match these to your placements or whichever subject you are currently learning about in lectures or SDL. There are just **so** many questions on there, it can easily get overwhelming if you don't filter.

- Start slowly: spend some proper time reading and working through the explanations below the answers, as these are often fantastic. When you are learning things for the first time, it's much better to work through ten questions thoroughly like this than to whizz through 100 without going into any detail.

- Adapt their explanations into your own notes, mind maps and flashcards. The authors of these sites often provide great mnemonics, tables and diagrams which present information in ways you hadn't previously thought of. By customising these into your own words and creating something more permanent, you can use them again and again to ensure the information sticks.

- Don't be demoralised by getting questions wrong: this is one of the most important ways to learn! Make sure you properly understand the explanation and concepts so you can get it right next time.

- If you really aren't getting the hang of a topic, be prepared to switch media and go back to your notes to try to understand it properly. People think that if they just keep doing enough online questions they will eventually get them right, but without the underlying knowledge you risk getting found out in exams when things are worded differently. Sometimes you need to take one step backwards before you can take two forwards.

- Pay attention to **how often** particular questions come up. If a topic comes up a lot, it's probably high yield and worth knowing about.

- Once you feel comfortable with the main concepts in your chosen subject you can start to build up volume and speed of online questions and add in multiple subjects at the same time, particularly in the run-up to exams. This is good for building up your pattern recognition, as you will start to spot recurring themes.

- But be wary of relying too heavily on one particular site for all your studying. Each has its own style of questioning and presenting information – this may not necessarily align with your medical school's exams, so you can easily get caught out by acclimatising to the wrong style.

The sheer volume of questions available online makes it very tempting to just mindlessly click through hundreds of them. Instead, narrow your field, go slowly, integrate the explanations with your other learning resources and make sure you actually understand the concepts properly. Only then should you start to build up your speed and quantity of questions.

### 3.3.5 The *BMJ*

If you haven't done so already, your first clinical year is a good time to check out all the great student-friendly articles available from the **British Medical Journal** (**BMJ**). Until very recently they published a stand-alone version called the **Student BMJ**, but at the time of writing this appears to have been integrated into the main **BMJ** and no longer exists as a separate entity. But not to worry, as you can still access loads of stuff at: www.bmj.com/student. These articles are pitched at a nice level for UK medical students and cover a huge range of topics from clinical subjects to OSCE tips, current affairs and medical politics. This a nice stepping stone to the proper grown-up medical journals which, in my view, are still rather intimidating at this stage! We'll discuss them in **Section 4.3.3**.

### 3.3.6 Patient information leaflets

A surprisingly under-utilised resource are those patient information leaflets which you find in wall-racks in hospital clinics and general practices. If you find yourself sitting around waiting for clinic to start, then these are a great thing to pick up and read as an entry-level introduction to a subject. Admittedly some are better written than others, but if you do find a good one you can get a superb overview of a disease or treatment in under ten minutes, written in plain English which you can easily understand!

Use patient information leaflets to prepare for OSCE stations in which you have to explain something to a patient. Consider the sorts of words and phrases the authors use, how they avoid jargon and articulate concepts clearly in layman's terms, and which pieces of information they have decided are most important to highlight to patients. This is a great exercise to help boost those vital communication skills.

### 3.3.7 Summary

In this section, we have looked at some resources to help you survive your first clinical year. The key points are:

- Start moving away from 'pure science' resources to those that include investigations, diagnosis and management.
- Get a small pocket-sized textbook to carry around on placements.
- Lecture slides are still useful but less essential than in previous years.
- If in doubt about which topics to study, ask yourself: would an FY1 need to know this?
- Download a few key apps and check out the many great websites available.
- Be smart in your use of online question banks instead of aimlessly trudging through thousands of questions without taking anything in.
- Check out the *BMJ*'s student-focused content for pointers on clinical placements, OSCEs and more.
- Nick a selection of patient information leaflets if you get the chance.

## 3.4 Clinical placements

Day one of clinical placements is when sh*t gets real. Torn from the comfortable bubble of university life, you are now thrown onto busy wards, into clinics, general practices and operating theatres. You have to talk to real patients, try to make sense of their problems, and understand what is being done to them and why. You'll witness the best of humanity and the worst, encounter death and misery perhaps for the first time, experience great times and bad, and see and smell things you never imagined possible (and that's just in your own pants).

Clinical placements can be scary but they are also tremendously exciting. This environment is where you will likely be spending the majority of your career, so it's important to get comfortable and confident with it. The first thing to note is that clinical placements provide a very different learning environment to the comfy seats and constant coffee supply of your medical school. See **Table 3.3** for some of the pros and cons of clinical placements. We'll explore these themes in more detail throughout this chapter.

**Table 3.3: The pros and cons of clinical placements compared to the university environment**

| Pros | Cons |
|---|---|
| • Learning from real patients with real histories, signs and symptoms | • Real patients are 'messy' – they have multiple diagnoses and don't fit into the neat boxes you learned from textbooks; this can be challenging at first |
| • Some patients *love* talking to medical students | • Some patients *hate* talking to medical students |
| • Getting to know doctors and observe them at work | |
| • Immense variety and flexibility | • Doctors are very busy and won't always have time to teach you |
| • Infinite learning opportunities | |
| • Observing events first-hand and seeing how cases develop over time | • Less structure – it isn't always obvious where you should be and what you should be doing |
| • Opportunities to get stuck in and practise your clinical, communication and procedural skills | • Sometimes you'll feel like you're wasting your time or getting in the way |
| • You can actually make a positive difference for patients | • Potential to get grilled/interrogated/shouted at/ made to feel stupid |
| • Start to shape your career ideas and get excited to become a doctor | • You can actually make things worse for patients |
| | • You might witness bad things which put you off a career in medicine |

## 3.4.1 Top tips for surviving clinical placements

Right from day one of your first clinical year, here are 14 things you can do to make the most of your placements:

1.  If you are given any choice in the matter, try to pick smaller hospitals, district generals and those with a strong teaching culture. You'll generally receive more attention and learn a lot more than at massive inner-city hospitals where everything is more crowded and everyone is busier. The quality of your experience can vary enormously between locations: speak to students in the years above for suggestions about which hospitals to go for and which to avoid.

2.  Carry a pocket-sized notebook to jot down all the conditions you encounter and the topics you need to research later. Look these up as soon as you get the chance, while they're still fresh in your

mind. Also note down memorable experiences and patients you encountered and the main things you learned each day. Look back over these at the end of each day and week to reinforce and consolidate your learning.

3. Use your pocket-sized textbook to quickly look things up while you are on placement, or just to leaf through during quiet moments. This looks much more professional than using your phone (sure, you might be reading the latest clinical trial in the *Lancet*, but people will probably assume you're checking Facebook).

4. Be prepared to 'play dumb' sometimes. You can learn absolutely LOADS by using phrases like "I'm sorry but I don't understand – would you mind explaining it to me?" or "This is probably a silly question, but …" or "I haven't learned about this condition yet – can we talk about it when we get a chance?"

5. Never be afraid to cry or feel sad. Once you start spending time with real patients, you will see some deeply upsetting things and hear some awful, tragic stories. Patients you've got to know may pass away, or suffer in ways you can't bear to witness. Don't bottle up your feelings: talk to friends, family, a tutor or a professional and learn how to recognise and process your feelings. I cried as a student and I've cried as an FY1: it's a natural, appropriate reaction to some situations and there is absolutely no shame in it whatsoever.

6. Really focus on improving your time management skills. Clinical placements are a lot more self-directed than teaching blocks, so it's a great opportunity to practise the essential skills discussed in *Section 2.6*. Make active decisions about how to spend your time: learn to be present when there's lots going on, and to sneak away when there's not. You'd be surprised how many people get this the wrong way round! And be flexible: if there is something interesting happening on your free afternoon and you think you'll get good teaching, then go along and take another half day off instead. It's unlikely anyone will notice or care, and you can justify it if they do.

7. Seek out informal teaching opportunities, as well as formal. You will need both types on clinical placements. Informal teaching tends to happen later in the day when people are a little less busy. For example, if a junior doctor seems enthusiastic to teach you but is rushed off their feet, ask them when would be a more suitable time and make an effort to come back and find them later.

8.  Learn to love clinical teaching fellows. These are usually trainees who have landed a temporary teaching post as part of their training, so they are highly motivated to teach students and have got dedicated time set aside to do so. They were universally fantastic in my experience, and you should attend any and every session they offer!

9.  Don't limit yourself by profession or seniority. Medicine is very hierarchical, and it is tempting to assume you should be learning from those at the top. But in fact you can learn from absolutely anyone at any time: I can recall amazing teaching I received on placements from FY1s, pharmacists, patients, nurses, midwives, physiotherapists and even other medical students. If someone is a good teacher and willing to spend time with you then you should grab that opportunity, whoever they are.

10. Forge human connections. Hospitals are extremely busy places, and most people are just trying to get their job done to the best of their abilities. Teaching students is probably not a core part of that job, so it's something you will have to 'earn'. You will find this **much** easier if you are polite and friendly, introduce yourself, smile and appear interested and enthusiastic. Once you have made a connection with someone you can chat to them, ask questions, and before you know it they're actually teaching you stuff.

11. Perfect your poker face. Whether showing you their oozing scrotal wound or explaining a bizarre sexual practice, patients will often shock and surprise you when you least expect it. Try to remain calm and non-judgemental at all times (***Figure 3.2***).

12. OMG WTF with the TLAs? Medicine is absolutely awash with acronyms – to the point where it even has its own in-joke (TLA stands for Three Letter Acronym). Whether it's NAI or PCI, TOF or PPI, get yourself into the habit of noting them down and working out what they mean, and eventually you'll start to understand what everyone is on about. And watch out for duplication: ASD can be autism spectrum disorder or atrial septal defect; ED can be emergency department or erectile dysfunction; RA can be right atrium, room air or rheumatoid arthritis, and so on. Be warned!

13. Feign interest. Hopefully your placements are interesting and enjoyable, but even during boring stretches there is still value in trying to look engaged and switched on. A great way to do this is to keep asking questions, even if you secretly don't give a toss about the answers. Just think of something reasonably intelligent to ask

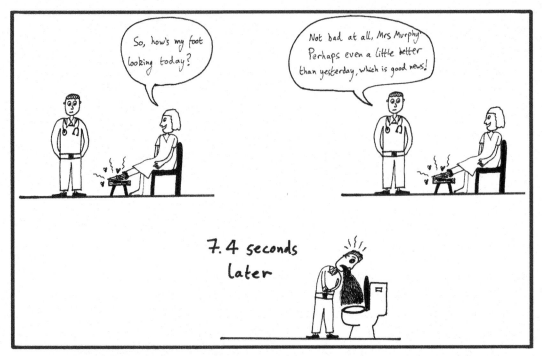

**Figure 3.2: Clinical placements are a good time to start perfecting your poker face.** You will need this as a doctor!

whenever you sense a chance. This will create a good impression, which greatly increases your odds of getting teaching on other subjects which you do enjoy.

14. Develop a thick skin. To quote the inspirational words given to us by a junior doctor at St George's, in an introductory lecture to becoming an FY1: "Some people are just knobs. Get used to it." Sadly she was right: no matter how keen, polite and friendly you are, there will always be the odd person who is horrible to you, particularly during your medical student and junior doctor years. Such behaviour is unacceptable and I'm not condoning it for one second, but I would strongly encourage you not to waste your valuable energy and time getting upset about it. These people often have their own issues and are just taking out their frustrations on someone lower down the food chain. Do not let them beat you down, because they are simply not worth damaging your studies and mental health for. Try to avoid them as best you can and channel your efforts into being a good person who can rise above it.

(An important caveat about this last point: I am talking about the sort of low-level unpleasantness which can be tolerated without lasting repercussions.

You will definitely encounter it and I think it helps if you are prepared for it. But of course there are limits: if unpleasant behaviour ever crosses a line into manifestly unprofessional conduct, abuse or bigotry, you should always discuss it with a senior or someone at the medical school. It is vital to look after yourself and not suffer in silence. You can also potentially do a great service to patients and your colleagues by speaking up, as someone who is horrible or unprofessional to medical students might be acting out in other, potentially serious ways too.)

## 3.4.2 Medical placements

Placements in your first clinical year are usually divided into medicine and surgery, and you will typically do at least one of each. We'll address both of these placements in turn to look at how you can get the most out of them.

At this early stage of your education, medical schools try to put you into busy, broad, generalist departments where you can get exposure to a wide range of patients and conditions. So on medical placements, you are typically attached to a ward covering one of the core specialties such as respiratory, gastroenterology or renal medicine. Alternatively, you might find yourself on a general medical ward, care of the elderly or the acute medical unit – all of which will give you great exposure to an enormous range of conditions.

Of course every hospital and every department is different, but there are some common themes. Notably the structure of the day, which tends to go something like *Figure 3.3*. The times will vary but the main thing to note is that the ward round is king on medical placements: it is the main event of the day, and sets the tone for everything else that happens later on. So as a student, you will inevitably spend a lot of time on ward rounds, and will probably be expected to attend them most days. For this reason, it's worth us taking a detailed look at them so you will know what to expect.

> Ward rounds are the main event of the day on medical placements. They are not always enjoyable for medical students, but there is no escaping them so try to extract as much from them as you can.

**KEY POINT**

### Ward rounds

The first thing you probably ought to know is: what actually happens on a ward round? At a basic level, this is when the medical team physically goes around the ward from bed to bed and sees all the patients. This might be all together, or the team might split up and see patients separately, depending

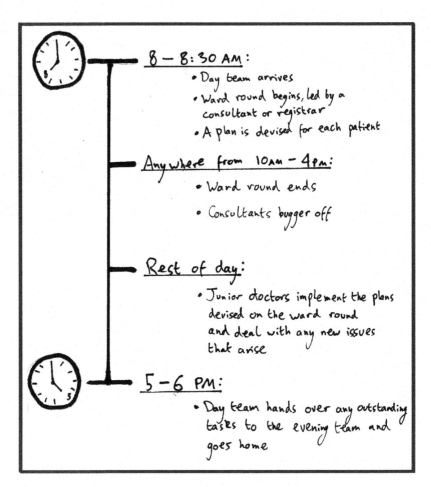

**8 – 8:30 AM:**
- Day team arrives
- Ward round begins, led by a consultant or registrar
- A plan is devised for each patient

**Anywhere from 10am – 4pm:**
- Ward round ends
- Consultants bugger off

**Rest of day:**
- Junior doctors implement the plans devised on the ward round and deal with any new issues that arise

**5 – 6 PM:**
- Day team hands over any outstanding tasks to the evening team and goes home

**Figure 3.3: The typical structure of the day on a medical ward.**

on staffing and other factors. It's often the **only** time a patient will get to see their doctors each day. But ward rounds are about much more than just **seeing** patients – really they are where the whole intellectual exercise of medicine takes place, condensed into a short window. To explain what I mean, let's break down the whole process that (in theory, anyway) the team goes through for each patient they see on the round (**Box 3.2**).

It might seem blindingly obvious that this is what ward rounds are all about. But I honestly can't remember anyone ever properly explaining this to me at medical school and I really wish they had! It's a classic example of assumed knowledge – the whole process of ward rounds is so deeply ingrained for doctors that they forget they ever didn't know it, and just assume that you know it too. But it wasn't until final year that I really felt comfortable with ward rounds and knew what was going on. Until then, I endured plenty of tedious mornings traipsing around the ward as a

**So what the hell actually happens on ward rounds?**

Here are nine steps that, in theory at least, the team will run through for every patient.

1. Discuss the patient's background, what brought them into hospital, what happened when they got there and what diagnosis they received.
2. Look at the patient's observations, fluid balance and any other relevant documentation from nurses, physios, and so on.
3. Look at results of blood tests, imaging and any other relevant investigations.
4. Review what medications and treatments have been given so far.
5. Ask the patient how they are today and whether any new issues have arisen since the previous day.
6. Revisit any parts of the history that are unclear and gather any other useful information from the patient.
7. Examine the patient.
8. Integrate **all of the above** information to come up with a diagnosis, or confirm that the existing diagnosis is still appropriate, and a plan of action for how the patient will be treated over the next 24 hours.
9. Explain the plan to the patient and write it clearly in the notes, so that everyone knows what needs to be done next.

Box 3.2

passive, uninvolved observer with little clue what the frick was going on. It is natural to feel this way – I suspect most medical students would rank ward rounds pretty low on their list of enjoyable learning activities. I hope that by demystifying the process you can start to find them a little more engaging.

The first issue, which you will spot very quickly, is that ward rounds are **enormously** variable in style, speed and content. The schema in **Box 3.2** is an **ideal** situation for what **should** happen every time a patient is seen on a round, but the reality is often extremely different! Some patients will get 30 minutes with the team; others will get 30 seconds. Sometimes you'll start washing your hands and realise the team has already seen the next patient before you've even dried off. And of course the structure gets heavily customised: you might be surprised when no one examines the patient, but actually some patients don't really need to be examined every day, so step 7 can be safely skipped. There might not be any investigations to review, so step 3 gets skipped, or the observations are unremarkable so step 2 gets reduced to the FY1 muttering "obs stable".

This variation in speed and content is partly explained by time pressures and fluctuations in workload, such as the number and complexity of patients

**KEY POINT**

> The enjoyableness of ward rounds for medical students depends heavily on who is leading them. Some consultants will teach you enthusiastically for three hours straight and buy you coffee at the end; others will completely ignore you or worse, appear positively irritated by your presence.

that need to be seen that day. But there is also a lot of personality that goes into ward rounds, which has a big impact on how enjoyable medical students find them. Every consultant has their own style: some simply *love* to teach, and will actively engage with you, get you to examine patients and keep you involved throughout the entire ward round. Others, sadly, will barely acknowledge your presence. They're not bad people, they just don't see ward rounds in that way: their priority is to patients, not students.

> **So as a learning experience, ward rounds are hit and miss: at their best, they're absolutely brilliant; at their worst, you'll wish you hadn't bothered getting out of bed.**

Unfortunately you are powerless to change consultants' style, but there are lots of things you can do to improve your enjoyment of ward rounds, particularly in the early years of med school. Check out my general pointers from **Section 3.4.1,** as lots of them will apply to ward rounds; particularly asking lots of questions, using a small textbook to look things up on the spot, and jotting down topics to research later. See **Box 3.3** for more top tips.

With ward rounds, as with any activity at medical school, keep asking yourself whether you are actually learning anything. If the rounds are fantastic and you are learning a lot, as is very often the case, I implore you to keep showing up, being attentive and guzzling up the information and skills that will maximise your chances of success. On the flip side, if the rounds suck as a learning experience and you can safely avoid them, then do! Find other activities and ways to get the most out of your placement. More on this later.

**Top tips for getting the most out of ward rounds**

Box 3.3

- Always try to get your own copy of the patient list before starting the round. This is absolutely essential for keeping track of what's going on: ward rounds are rubbish when you don't even know who the patients are and what diagnoses they have!
- Try to arrive ten minutes early and introduce yourself to the doctors. This makes you appear polite and enthusiastic, which greatly increases the chances of people engaging with you. If you show up when the round is already under way you may find yourself at the back, being ignored. I speak from bitter experience!
- Get involved and look interested: stay as close to the front as you can, ask questions, write notes and smile at patients. This will make you feel like part of the team. If a patient has clinical signs, ask if you can quickly examine to check that you can see/hear/feel it for yourself.
- Don't panic if the ward round feels overwhelming. That's normal. It is very ambitious to hope to understand everything, so just pick a few high-yield topics you want to focus on and save the rest for later.
- If you are suffering from information overload, try using the schema in *Box 3.2* to focus on areas of practice rather than diseases. For example, you could pick one day to focus on step 3 – interpreting blood tests and imaging. This will help break the ward round into chunks and improve your pattern recognition to boot.
- Infectious patients are put into side rooms for isolation, and you might be required to don gloves, aprons and masks before entering. If so, *practise* doing this in an afternoon when no one is looking – particularly the plastic aprons, which are fiddly as hell. I personally have been defeated by them many times during ward rounds!
- If the ward is using paper notes, practise skimming through patients' folders during quiet times when no one else is using them. Work out where the drug charts and obs charts are kept and how to extract the key information quickly. These folders are tricky to navigate so it is good to practise in a low-pressure situation.
- Don't rush to judgement. You will witness some poor practice and diabolical bedside manner on ward rounds, particularly the ones conducted at breakneck speed. Of course that's not cool, but try to resist the temptation to write doctors off based solely on their ward rounds. There is usually more going on 'behind the scenes' than you are aware of. The ward round is just a small snapshot of the patient's care so don't immediately assume the worst.
- Try to enjoy yourself. Whether you realise it or not, as a medical student you are in a privileged position in that you get to attend ward rounds purely for your own learning without any genuine expectation of you. For the rest of the team, they can be highly pressurised situations. This is perhaps something that can only be appreciated with retrospect once you become an FY1, but trust me you've got a pretty cushy gig!

## Aftermath

At some point, once all the patients have been seen, the ward round will come to an end. Sometimes this is extremely abrupt, signalled only by the doctor walking off (classically a surgeon), leaving you adrift and unsure what to do with yourself. In other, more collegiate teams, the round might end with a 'board round' or 'huddle', which involves everyone getting together around the patient whiteboard for a quick run-through of all the patients on the ward. Whichever doctor saw each patient on the round that morning will provide a brief update on their care, and ensure that everyone on the team knows what needs to be done next.

At this point, it becomes important to appreciate that the ward round serves different purposes for different members of the team. The more senior the doctor, the more the round is about performing that intellectual exercise of medicine we discussed above – about devising the plans and leading the team. The more junior the doctor, the more the round is about simply implementing the plans which have been devised by the leader. So for the most junior doctors of the lot, the FY1s and FY2s, the entire ward round essentially boils down to a series of tasks they need to get through, known as 'jobs'. Examples might include 'order chest X-ray for bed 22', 'take blood from bed 4' or 'refer bed 17 for an orthopaedic opinion'. The juniors will usually write all these jobs down on a piece of paper entitled 'jobs list' with a little box next to each one, which they fill in once it's been completed (**Figure 3.4**).

> **TOP TIP**
>
> During the ward round, try to figure out who's who and observe their different roles. In a nutshell: senior doctors *make* the plans; juniors *implement* them.

The reason this is important for you to appreciate as a medical student is because it has a direct bearing on what you do once the round ends and who you are going to hang out with for the rest of your day. Unless specifically invited to do so, you **do not** follow the consultant and attempt to keep discussing NICE guidelines, Light's criteria or the significance of T-wave inversion, no matter how enthusiastically they discussed this with you during the round. It is an established convention that consultants leave the ward after completing the round – I don't know where they go or what they do, but I do know that following them would be a form of social suicide. Instead, you either seize the opportunity to sneak away unnoticed, or turn your attention to the FY1s and SHOs and figure out what to do next.

There is usually a short flurry of activity immediately after the ward round while the juniors create a jobs list and strategise about how best to

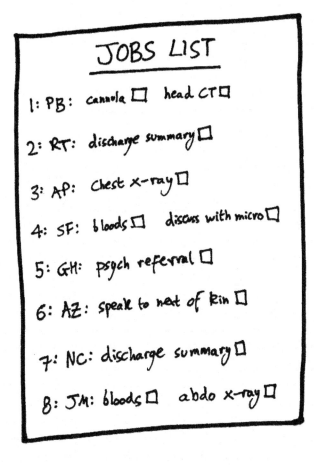

JOBS LIST

1: PB: cannula ☐   head CT☐

2: RT: discharge summary☐

3: AP: chest x-ray☐

4: SF: bloods ☐   discuss with micro☐

5: GH: psych referral ☐

6: AZ: speak to next of kin ☐

7: NC: discharge summary☐

8: JM: bloods☐   abdo x-ray☐

**Figure 3.4: Example of a junior doctor's jobs list.** Patients are listed by bed number and initials, to protect anonymity, with the outstanding tasks listed next to them. And yes: we still write these out on paper. And yes: I know it's 2019.

tackle it in the time that remains. You'll need to take a back seat for this, so either grab some lunch and come back later, or wait patiently for them to finish. Once the dust settles, you will be entering a twilight zone we will refer to as 'unstructured ward time'.

## Unstructured ward time

On medical placements, there can be a lot of time when you are supposed to be on the ward but do not have any specific activities on your timetable. For many students, the big question is whether to show up at all during these periods: we will address this in **Section 3.4.6**. But for now, let's assume you do attend the ward after rounds have finished – what are you supposed to do with yourself? Realistically, on medical placements, there are three options: clerk patients, perform procedures or get informal teaching (**Figure 3.5**).

Of these, the first two are art forms in themselves – both are lifelong skills requiring immense amounts of practise (we will discuss them in **Sections 3.4.4**, **3.4.9**, **4.5.2** and **4.5.6**). Informal teaching from junior doctors is often

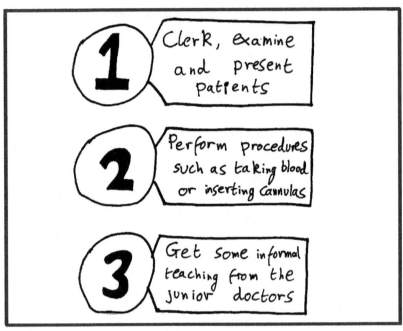

**Figure 3.5: Your main options for how to spend unstructured time on the ward during medical placements.**

harder to get but is extremely valuable so it is well worth putting in the effort (see **Box 3.4**). You can't just waltz in and out of the ward and expect it to happen on demand: you'll need to use all the behaviours and concepts we have discussed so far, and then the informal teaching will usually follow on by itself. It tends to happen fairly spontaneously, so you will need to be flexible and patient and wait for the right opportunity to present itself. Sometimes this means popping to the canteen or library for a couple of hours and coming back later.

A great way to decide your strategy for unstructured ward time is to look at the doctors' jobs lists once the round finishes and ask one of the juniors whether there is anything you can help them with. This makes you seem helpful and proactive, rather than someone who is just hanging around waiting to be told what to do. There will usually be a lot of paperwork and administrative tasks on the jobs lists, such as making referrals, chasing test results, requesting scans and writing discharge summaries. **Do not** get roped into doing these at this stage of medical school – that's what final year is for, and until then they are not a good use of your time. Stick to procedures and activities that involve patient contact. They shouldn't really be asking you to do admin at this stage of your studies, so it's fine to politely decline if there is no educational value in it for you.

**Top tips for securing informal teaching from junior doctors on the wards**

Box 3.4

1. 'Earn it' by being enthusiastic, interested, punctual and professional. If you look like you don't give a sh*t, then no one is going to waste their time on you.
2. Use people skills: be polite and friendly, introduce yourself and make an effort to remember doctors' names and roles. This establishes a connection from which you can initiate conversation.
3. Try to ask specific questions, preferably linked to a patient to demonstrate interest. For example: "I noticed we started Mr Green on furosemide today. I'm not too familiar with that drug yet, can I ask you some questions about it?" This will get you better teaching on diuretics and fluid balance than just saying: "Can you teach me about diuretics and fluid balance?"
4. Other potential conversation starters include following up on things you saw or heard on the ward round, asking to look at imaging, presenting a patient you have clerked or doing a procedure. For example: "I've taken those bloods you asked for. I was just wondering why we are monitoring LFTs in this patient, would you mind if we quickly looked at their previous results together?"
5. Once you've opened a conversation with one of the juniors, stay engaged, ask questions and jot down notes if they say something useful. They are much more likely to keep going if they feel like you are getting something out of it.
6. Most junior doctors instinctively *want* to teach you, but are limited by how busy and/or stressed they are. Be aware and sensitive to this: if it's not a good time, don't push it. If they ask you to come back later at a specific time then you should actually do so because it's rude not to, and you might get some great teaching when they're less busy. If you get a non-specific fob-off, on the other hand, then they probably aren't keen to teach and you can safely slink off.
7. When you do get informal teaching, thank them and say you found it helpful. Chances are they'll be happy to do it again sometime.

**Remember that the jobs list represents the juniors' workload for the rest of the day. So if it is huge then they are going to be very busy and probably won't have much time to teach you. If it is short, that might be a good day to stick around and try your luck.**

You should start to get a general feel for this from how busy the ward round is and by sensing everyone's stress levels afterwards! Don't be offended if everyone is too busy to teach you after the ward round – just

> **TOP TIP** Take a peek at the doctors' jobs lists after the ward round to help decide whether it's worth sticking around to try to get some informal teaching or best to make yourself scarce.

go do something else and try again another day. On the plus side, they'll also be too busy to notice or care when you sneak off from the ward.

## Clinics

Outpatient clinics are likely to figure prominently in your timetable for medical placements, and you will typically be expected to attend at least one a week. At this stage, you are essentially just there as an observer (as opposed to penultimate and final year when you might start seeing patients on your own), although you may be invited to examine patients under supervision, ask them questions or do the odd procedure. As with most of medical school, no one really tells you what to expect from clinics or how to get the most out of them, so I'll try to talk you through it.

The first thing to note is that – just like ward rounds – clinics are **extremely** variable as a learning experience. At their best, I attended clinics where the consultant kept me constantly involved with questions, teaching and explanations, introduced me to every patient like I was an integral part of the team, got me to examine everyone and spent half an hour with me at the end going over everything I'd seen and learned. At their worst, I've sat in the corner being completely ignored for three hours while patients came and went, barely even registering my presence. This can be a lonely, frustrating and demoralising experience – not to mention a lousy use of your time.

Some doctors occupy the extremes of this spectrum: either natural born teachers who love having students with them, or grumpy sods who would genuinely prefer you to bugger off and leave them alone. But the majority sit somewhere in the middle: they are keen to teach you in theory but are usually busy, sometimes stressed and always focused on the patient first and foremost. They therefore get distracted from teaching, and can easily lapse into ignoring you by accident. These are the ones where your attitude can make all the difference between a positive and negative learning experience.

See **Box 3.5** for some specific tips on how to go about this.

**If you remain active, engaged and interested, the doctor will keep remembering you are there and will be constantly reminded to talk to you and teach you. If you sit silently in the corner, showing no interest or enthusiasm, you're making it too easy for them to ignore you – and they almost certainly will.**

**Eight top tips for getting the most from outpatient clinics**     Box 3.5

1. Aim to sit in with doctors who you know are enthusiastic teachers. There can be a lot of competition between students for these spots, so you may need to sign up in advance or get there early!
2. Always introduce yourself clearly and confidently and ask politely if it's okay to sit in on the clinic. Appear enthusiastic and interested in the subject or disease.
3. Have some ideas about what you want to learn from that particular clinic and state these up front if possible (remember it's fine to play dumb!) For example: "I've been learning about diabetes this week but I find all the different medications confusing, so was hoping to learn a little more about them."
4. Try to sit close to the action so you feel involved in the consultation and can easily ask questions without shouting. Positioning your chair in the furthest corner is the first step towards being ignored.
5. Stay enthusiastic and ask the doctor as many questions as you can without being overbearing or interrupting consultations. This can be a delicate balancing act! But each time a patient leaves the room you could gently try at least one question, or ask to quickly look at the relevant test results or imaging before the next patient enters.
6. Bring your small textbook so you can look up anything you are unclear about. Make notes to yourself and jot down the key points of any particularly memorable cases (anonymised, of course).
7. Aim to learn at least three things from any clinic you attend. Write these down immediately afterwards and look over them again while they are still fresh in your mind.
8. If you've tried all of the above and it really isn't going well, then make your excuses and leave rather than wasting your time. But don't just write off the whole morning or afternoon: go to the library for an hour instead and try a different approach to tackling the topic you had in mind.

Ultimately you may conclude you simply don't enjoy spending time in clinics at this stage of medical school. That's common and understandable, lots of students feel that way, but clinics are an integral part of medical practice so I'm afraid you can't give up on them altogether! If you only ever see inpatients on wards, you'll see only the sickest, most acute cases and end up with a very skewed view of how particular conditions are managed. To understand a disease properly, you also need to see people living with it on a daily basis, experiencing symptoms and side-effects and having small but important adjustments made to their treatment. Lots of the highest-yield conditions are managed predominantly in general practice and outpatient specialty clinics: diabetes, asthma, cancer, dementia and ischaemic heart disease, to name but a few. You can learn an absolutely huge amount from clinics so it really is worth persisting with them – even if you don't stay for the whole thing every time.

**KEY POINT**

Clinics can be hit and miss for medical students when you're purely observing. But when they're good they're extremely valuable for your learning and you should persist with them – I got some absolutely fantastic teaching there.

### 3.4.3 Surgical placements

Surgical placements, in my experience, can be the most tricky and daunting for medical students, particularly in the early years. The adage that 'you get out what you put it in' can be applied to most of medical school, but it is **especially** true for surgical placements. No one is going to hold your hand and walk you through it: you will need to show initiative, resilience and flexibility, and in many cases you will have to work to 'earn' good teaching and experiences. But when you do succeed, you'll find the teaching is some of the best you receive in all of medical school and the experiences some of the most inspirational. Persevere!

The first thing to do when you start in surgery is to get your head around the who, when and where. Start by finding out the consultant surgeons' names, what they specialise in, which days they are in theatre and clinics, when departmental meetings take place, and where the wards and operating theatres are (**Figure 3.6**). Your timetable and handbook are the obvious starting point, but I always found there were plenty of gaps and outdated information you had to fill in for yourself by asking staff members, the last bunch of students, and even Googling names and

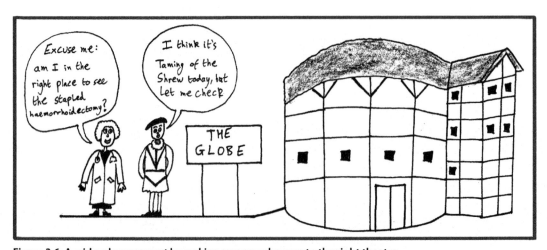

Figure 3.6: Avoid embarrassment by making sure you show up to the right theatre.

departments. Next, try to figure out who the registrars, SHOs and FY1s are, and roughly what their responsibilities and working patterns are. It can take a few days to establish all of this but, once you do, it makes it so much easier to slot yourself in. You'll soon realise that certain people are great for certain activities at certain times – you just need to work out who and what these are so you can target them effectively!

> Spend a bit of time at the start of surgery placements figuring out who's who and when and where everything happens. This will make it much easier to slot yourself in.

At the beginning, you might assume that a surgical placement is all about being in the operating theatre but in fact there are several different ways to spend your time. Let's consider all the different activities that occur on a surgical firm and how you can get the most out of them.

## Surgical ward rounds

Ward rounds in surgery are usually much more rapid than on medical placements and it can be extremely hard to keep up! By the time you've worked out what procedure patient 1 had and why, they've already moved onto patient 5 and you are none the wiser. Interaction with patients can be ultra-brief and unenlightening, while documentation may be as minimalist as: "Obs stable, afebrile. Abdomen soft. Plan: continue." And because everything is happening so fast, everyone has less time to teach and explain things to you, so it can feel alienating at times (**Figure 3.7**).

> Surgical ward rounds are *rapid* and you will struggle to follow everything. You will often have to come back and examine patients later if you are to get anything out of the experience.

For these reasons, I wouldn't recommend attending surgical ward rounds every day at this early stage of medical school as you will swiftly get bored! Two or three times per week is probably reasonable, assuming you can get away with it. You can go to theatre and clinics on the other mornings, or do some SDL then head to the ward later. If you can get away with choosing which days you attend rounds, try to go along on days after attending theatres, so that you can see the same patients you saw operated on, understand how they are recovering and whether they developed any complications. And if you have no choice but to attend rounds every day, well, the good news is they are usually over quite quickly!

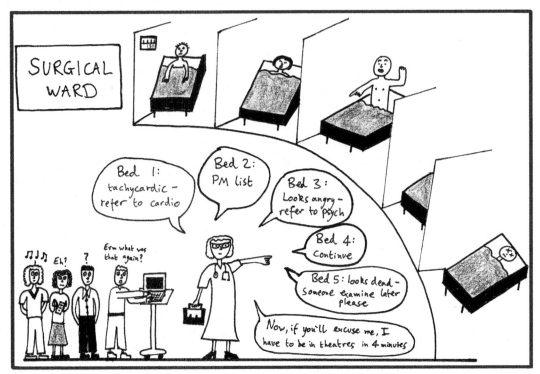

**Figure 3.7: Surgical ward rounds can be extremely fast and you may not learn very much as an observer.** Try to come back later to examine patients, take histories and discuss cases in more detail with the junior doctors.

**TOP TIP**

Don't be late for a surgical ward round. You'll show up and find you've missed it.

During the ward round, do keep trying to engage and ask questions where possible, using all the tips in **Box 3.5**. However, in surgery you may swiftly realise it's not appropriate to ask lots of questions as you don't want to slow everyone down. If so, your best bet is just to tag along quietly, observe as best you can and make a list of interesting-sounding patients and topics to look up. Come back later to clerk and examine these patients, read their notes and ask questions to the FY1s and SHOs when they have a little more free time later in the day. They should be sympathetic if you say: "I had a couple of questions from this morning's ward round but it was all a bit rushed, is it okay if I ask you now?"

## Operating theatres

Attending operating theatres for the first time can be extremely exciting but also a little nerve-racking. Personally I found the operating theatre quite an intimidating environment to begin with as a medical student. There are

> The operating theatre can be a very intimidating environment for medical students to begin with. This feeling will hopefully pass as you grow in confidence and start to establish how everything works.

**KEY POINT**

so many people buzzing around, all with very specific roles, operating like cogs in a huge and well-oiled machine. And then there's you – an outsider with no particular job, not sure where to stand, what to do or what to say. You don't know what most of the equipment is but you're not sure who you can ask about it, and you sure as hell know you'd better not touch anything for fear of breaking sterility. There's also the fact that a real, actual life is at stake in front of you, and you desperately don't want to distract anyone or do anything that could jeopardise the patient's safety. And if all that wasn't enough, there are often huge personalities and egos to contend with and a rigid hierarchy that trumps any other area of medicine. Unfortunately, these factors can all create the sense that your best strategy is just to keep shtum, avoid pissing anyone off and fade quietly into the background. Which is a real shame because that's not a great strategy for learning or getting inspired to pursue a career in surgery.

**The good news is these feelings will pass: I found my experiences in the operating theatre got better and better each year, and by final year I realised I was actually enjoying myself! You just need to manage your expectations, be patient and view your surgery placements as one long, gradual process – you are not going to be scrubbing in and clamping vessels on day one, but someday you just might.**

Based on extensive trial and error, here are my top tips to help you get the most out of your time in theatre:

- **Plan ahead:** decide in advance which days you want to go to theatre, find out who the surgeons are and see if you can get a copy of their operating lists the day before. Introduce yourself to the consultant or registrar beforehand and ask if it is okay to join them in theatre.

> Manage your expectations when it comes to spending time in the operating theatre. To begin with, you will spend a lot of time standing at the back feeling useless. But as you progress through the years, you will get more opportunities to scrub in and feel like you are actually learning and getting involved.

**TOP TIP**

Of course they are obliged to say yes! But asking is polite, makes a good impression and helps to build some rapport before you show up. Make sure to check exactly where and when you should arrive. And choose your procedures wisely: if it starts at 3 p.m. and is likely to last for seven hours, involves super-specialised techniques which will never come up in your exams, or is being performed by a surgeon notorious for bollocking medical students, I'd suggest you steer clear. By just blindly showing up without any prior research, you are risking any/all of the above.

- **Always try to meet the patient first:** modern surgery has evolved to be totally dehumanising: if you walk into a theatre when the patient is already anaesthetised and covered by drapes, you'll find the entire complexity of their being has been reduced to an exposed slab of skin through which the surgeon can access their organs, muscles and vessels. That's helpful for the person who has to cut into them, but rubbish for the student who also needs to learn about the patient and their disease. You'll find surgery so much more engaging and meaningful when you have met and clerked the patient beforehand, heard about how their disease presented and changed over time, and examined them thoroughly. You're also more likely to get dibs on scrubbing in and assisting if you actually know the patient! Most of the time they will be happy to chat to a medical student beforehand, and will like the idea of having a 'friendly face' in theatre with them.

- **Err on the early side:** better to show up early, meet the patient and surgeon then twiddle your thumbs for a bit than to show up when it's already under way and try introducing yourself to the surgeon from the back of the room. They tend not to like this very much! Showing up early also allows you to watch the patient being consented and prepped for surgery and to take part in the WHO checklist, which is great learning fodder. The checklist also provides an opportunity to introduce yourself, write your name on the whiteboard, make it feel like you are part of the team, and learn about everyone else's roles. This often involves an earlier start than you are used to but this maximises your morning, meaning you can head off guilt-free in the afternoon.

- **Do some homework:** read up on the procedure and relevant anatomy beforehand. This will increase your interest levels and help you survive any grillings coming your way. I found it helpful to pick out the relevant Netter's anatomy flashcards the night before then go over them on the train that morning. Some surgeons have particular topics they like to grill all their students on – if you can find these out in advance, you'd be wise to have some answers ready (see **Box 3.6**).

> **Surgeons *love* grilling students on precise definitions of surgical terminology**
>
> Here are some classic examples to rote learn so you can effortlessly recall them in theatre.[2]
>
> - **Hernia:** the protrusion of an organ or tissue out of the body cavity in which it normally lies.
> - **Fistula:** an abnormal communication between two hollow organs, connecting two mucosa-lined surfaces, or between a hollow organ and the exterior.
> - **Abscess:** a localised collection of pus and necrotic tissue anywhere in the body, surrounded and walled off by damaged and inflamed tissues.
> - **Ileus:** intestinal obstruction.
> - **Ischaemia:** an inadequate flow of blood to a part of the body, caused by constriction or blockage of the blood vessels supplying it.
> - **Infarction:** the death of part or the whole of an organ that occurs when the artery carrying its blood supply is obstructed by a blood clot or embolus.
> - **Stoma:** the artificial opening of a tube (e.g. the colon or ileum) that has been brought to the abdominal surface.
> - **Slough:** dead tissue, such as skin, that separates from healthy tissue after inflammation or infection. (NB this is pronounced *sluff*, not like the town to the west of London.)

Box 3.6

- **Scrub in as often as possible:** at this stage of medical school you are likely to be watching from the back of the theatre, particularly if there are more senior students around. Nevertheless if you do get the opportunity to scrub in I suggest you grab it, as the action is far more engaging when you have a front row seat. Plus you are more likely to get some informal teaching and might even be asked to assist, which is super-exciting at first! The actual process of scrubbing in can be a bit scary but the best way to learn is by practising so you're better off taking the plunge sooner rather than later. Be open and admit that you've not done it many times before but are keen to learn – often there'll be a scrub nurse or operating department practitioner (ODP) who can help you out with the fiddly bits like the weird pirouette around that little cardboard tag.

- **Be nice to everyone:** no matter how badly you want to be a surgeon, don't fall into the trap of thinking they are the only people in the room who you can learn from. At this stage, pretty much everyone else in that theatre is more knowledgeable than you, and a little humility really can go a long way. Introduce yourself to all the auxiliary staff, smile and be polite, and you'll find people will be far more willing to explain things to you and help you out than if you completely ignore them while kissing the surgeon's bum at every opportunity.

- **Study the people and kit:** if you do find yourself at the back of the theatre and can't really follow the operation, focus instead on trying to work out who all the different people are and what all the equipment is for. Often you'll be able to have a quiet chat with a friendly ODP or nurse on the sidelines – be honest that this is all new to you and you'd love to ask some really dumb questions about what's going on. They're usually happy to answer, which can help you turn a long and pointless session into one where you at least learned something, even if it wasn't the topic you expected.

- **Adjust to surgical time:** time passes weirdly in surgery. You'll experience long boring stretches of absolutely nothing happening while everyone waits for the patient to arrive, then an intense flurry of activity while they are prepped and the operation gets under way. The procedure itself can whizz by if you are scrubbed in, or drag on forever if you're zoned out on the sidelines. Then another flurry while the patient is closed and taken to recovery, before time slows back to a crawl while everyone waits for the next one to show up (seriously, in between operations, you'll see some of the most highly skilled, highly paid people in the NHS sitting in the surgeons' lounge with their feet up doing the crossword, which is totally weird at first, **Figure 3.8**). Once you get used to this ebb and flow, you can start to work out when to speak up and when to stay quiet. For example, some surgeons love to teach during an operation but will bite your head off if you talk to them during their downtime in the lounge. Others will operate in near silence then come to life between procedures and start teaching you anatomy on the whiteboard.

- **Choose your moments wisely:** carry a small textbook to get you through the boring stretches at the back of the theatre, and make sure to perk up and look lively when things get interesting. Above all, use some common sense – if you've clerked the patient and think the registrar might be receptive to discussing the case with you, approach them during one of those quiet moments beforehand, not when they're scrubbed in and just about to open up the patient!

- **Befriend the anaesthetist:** patients will usually spend somewhere between five and 30 minutes in the anaesthetic room off to the side before going into the main operating theatre. This is time when you might otherwise be doing bugger all, particularly if your surgeon is the

---

2 *Oxford Concise Medical Dictionary*, 8th edition.

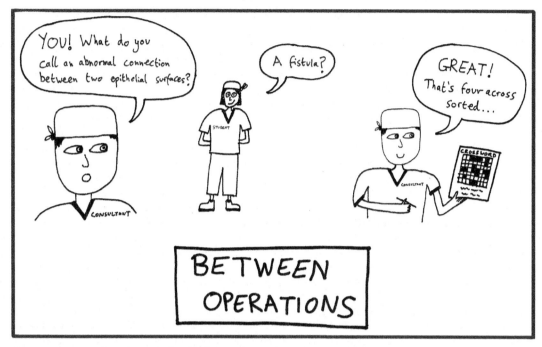

**Figure 3.8: As a student, it can be hard to know what to do with yourself in between operations.** Some surgeons will teach/grill you further, others will just ignore you and do the crossword. Take the opportunity to stretch your legs, drink water and go to the toilet, and bring some reading material to keep you going if all else fails.

sullen 'no chat between operations' type. If so, try saying hello to the anaesthetist and asking whether you can quietly pop yourself in the corner and observe their preparations. By and large, anaesthetists are a lovely bunch who are enthusiastic to teach medical students, even if you're not yet on an anaesthetics placement. Just explain that you feel anaesthesia is an equally important part of the patient's journey and you'd love to learn more about it. Before you know it they're teaching you physiology and pharmacology and getting you to insert cannulas. And if they say no then it's no harm done, and you can go back to watching the surgeon do the crossword.

• **Look after yourself:** in theatre, everyone is completely consumed by looking after the patient and doing their job properly, so your welfare is very low down their list of priorities. Make sure it remains high on yours: eat a good breakfast and caffeinate yourself before going to theatre, sit down when you get a chance, drink plenty of water and ensure you know exactly where the toilets are. You can be on your feet for a long time, which is tough if you're not used to it. Oh and wear a vest under your scrubs, because operating theatres are ***coooooooooooold***.

No matter how bored you might be at the back of the theatre, bear in mind that it could always be worse. One of my fellow FY1s was observing a gynaecological procedure as a student when one of the stirrups for elevating the patient's legs broke, and no replacement could be found. With the procedure already under way, and the patient's positioning being critical to its success, she was recruited to stand at the end of the bed with the patient's foot on her shoulder. She stood like that for well over an hour – acting as a glorified footrest for a leg that felt heavier and heavier – without so much as a short break. You'd be pretty glad to return to the back of the theatre after that!

## Unstructured ward time

This is perhaps the most neglected aspect of surgical placements by medical students, but there is a lot to be learned if you can find the right times and people. Early mornings tend to be very hectic with ward rounds, surgeons planning their operating lists and consenting patients, and juniors frantically working out what jobs need to be done. But if you head to surgical wards late morning or early afternoon it is usually much quieter, and a great time to practise clerking, examinations and procedures.

Consultants and registrars are likely to be in theatres at these times, so the SHOs and FY1s are in charge and you might be able to wangle a bit of informal teaching out of them, or at least present a patient and get some feedback. This is also a great time to boost your radiology and pathology knowledge by reviewing patients' scans and test results and asking someone to discuss them with you. You'll often be the only medical student around in the afternoons so people will be impressed with your enthusiasm (don't tell them you just got out of bed at midday and came straight to the ward).

**KEY POINT**

Afternoons on surgical wards are much quieter than mornings and are a great time to practise clerking, examination and procedures or get informal teaching from the juniors.

In surgery, as opposed to medicine, there is an even greater emphasis on physical signs and examination, so try to focus your ward learning and case presentations by getting hands-on wherever possible. Feel lumps, look at stomas, examine hernias and palpate transplanted kidneys – the more you see and do, the more you will build up your pattern recognition and boost your confidence. I'm not suggesting you completely neglect the communication side of things but believe me, when you are presenting a case to a surgeon they will be much more interested in the location and size of a lump than the patient's social situation or anxieties about the operation. I can still recall the bewildered look on a GI surgeon's face when a student told him exactly how many cats and dogs the patient had – this was totally irrelevant information!

> Really focus on improving your examination skills and recognition of physical signs during surgical placements. Surgeons are far more interested in these than your communication skills!

You can also use unstructured ward time to follow up on patients you have seen in clinic, A&E, pre-op assessment and theatres. Keep an eye on their progress so you can build up the whole picture of their condition: how did it present, how long did it take to diagnose, what tests and scans did they have, was there any medical management, how did the procedure itself go, were there any complications, when were they discharged and how were they followed up? This sort of information sticks in your brain much better than stuff learned from a textbook.

> Keep tabs on patients you have seen in operating theatres and surgical clinics to see how their case unfolded afterwards. Try to build up a complete picture of their condition and commit it to memory alongside their face and name. This will stick a lot better than abstract concepts learned from textbooks.

**TOP TIP**

## Surgical clinics

Surgical clinics can be even more hit and miss than medical clinics, as they are usually very busy without much time for teaching. I would therefore suggest avoiding clinics at the very beginning of surgical placements until you have established who's who. That way you can target the clinics with people you know to be good teachers – hopefully they will involve you and get you taking histories and examining patients. Remember that a surgeon's seniority and reputation don't always correlate to the learning experience for you as a student: registrars often run their own clinics and some are far more enthusiastic about teaching than consultants!

When clinics do go well, they are also a good environment to establish a connection with surgeons before attending the operating theatre. If you had good rapport during the clinic then at the end you can ask which days are best to join them in theatre, or whether they have any interesting cases coming up which you could observe. That way, assuming you do actually show up in theatre, they'll recognise you and hopefully engage with you much better than if they are seeing you there for the first time. By seeming genuinely interested in their work, you are greatly increasing the chances of getting some good teaching out of them!

**TOP TIP**

Try to choose specific clinics where you think the surgeon will be interested in teaching you and getting you to examine patients. Otherwise you can find yourself in the corner being ignored. Again.

## On calls

Some placements will give you the chance to shadow whichever member of the surgical team is on call for the shift, i.e. they are carrying the bleep and assessing any new referrals made to the team. Like clinics, you are one-on-one with that person so the quality of the experience is highly dependent on them and how much they want to engage with you. There's also luck of the draw in terms of how busy the shift is and what sort of referrals come in. But when the elements do come together this is a fantastic and much-overlooked learning opportunity, and I would strongly urge you to jump on it. I didn't get to do it until final year and I felt it was a real shame I hadn't done it earlier.

Why did I love on calls so much? Well mainly because there is huge variety: when I shadowed the general surgical SHO on call we were assessing a potential bowel obstruction in A&E one minute, then a post-surgical complication on an adult ward the next, then down to the paediatric ward for an opinion on a possible appendicitis, then to operating theatres to update the consultant surgeon. It was extremely busy but there was never a dull moment, and being on your feet and moving around keeps you much more awake and interested than sitting down in a clinic. I received a lot of informal teaching on these shifts and found I learned a lot. There is also the potential to actually help out the person you are shadowing (a rarity as a medical student!): they will usually have an ever-growing backlog of patients to see and, depending on your skill level and confidence, you can save them time by chipping in with jobs such as taking blood, or going off on your own to clerk the new patients.

**KEY POINT**

Shadowing an on-call surgeon can be a great learning experience: there is lots of variety and you will get to see patients presenting for the first time, often in acute situations requiring emergency surgery. If you only attend clinics and elective procedures, you will completely miss this aspect of surgery which would be a real shame.

Don't be deterred if shadowing an on-call isn't on your timetable at this stage of medical school. Just keep your ears to the ground: if someone you are on good terms with mentions they are on call next week, there is no harm in asking whether you can tag along at some point. You don't need to do the whole shift – even just a few hours at the beginning can be very informative. They might even welcome the company!

## Freestyle

Don't be constrained by your timetable or the activities listed above – you can learn a lot by showing some initiative and finding your own things to do. Got some downtime on a colorectal surgery placement? Go watch some colonoscopies or shadow the stoma nurse. On breast surgery? Visit the chemotherapy suite, attend a multidisciplinary team meeting (MDT) or observe some mammograms being performed. Essentially, anything that improves your wider understanding of the specialty is worth attending, even if it seems slightly tangential to the core activities on your firm. You don't need to stick around for hours, just long enough to understand the basics. As long as you introduce yourself properly and ask politely whether you can sit in, you will quickly find that anything is possible. And going off-piste in this way usually means you'll be the only medical student around, which can be vastly preferable to jostling for position in crowded clinics and theatres. The worst that can happen is you get turned away – you are very unlikely to get into trouble for showing initiative and attempting to carve out your own learning opportunities!

## Being adaptable

My final word on surgical placements reflects a common theme running through everything we have discussed in this section. It took me a long time to put my finger exactly on it, but it's perhaps best articulated as follows:

> **You will get the most out of surgery by adapting yourself to the placement, not expecting the placement to adapt to you.**

This might seem obvious but sadly it's a conclusion I have reached by observing countless students get it the wrong way round. In final year, for example, I was on a busy surgical firm where ward rounds began at 8 a.m. sharp, were conducted at breakneck speed and finished by 9.30 at the latest. As in any firm, the ward rounds were a very important part of the day, particularly for the FY1s and SHOs, as this allowed them to make job lists and to plan out their day. There were several third-year students on the firm and the doctors were quite relaxed about attendance: as long as each student showed their face a handful of times each week, no one was looking too closely at who showed up on which day.

Unfortunately there was one student who stands out in my mind as having completely missed the point. He would consistently show up to the doctors' office around 9.30–10 a.m. and say something like: "Hey guys, sorry I missed the ward round … any jobs I can do?" The FY1s would grunt some sort of acknowledgement, say no there was nothing to do just now, then get back to their paperwork and proceed to completely ignore him. He'd sit there for a while checking his phone and making small talk, then decide he'd had enough and drift off by 10.30 a.m., usually heading to the student common room or library and not returning to the ward until the next morning. I later overheard him complaining to a friend about the placement, questioning why he bothered showing up every morning when no one taught him anything or gave him any procedures to do. He felt it was a complete waste of his time.

I sort of understand his perspective: yes it's a very early start to get there for 8 a.m., and he felt his efforts to attend were going unrewarded as he wasn't learning anything. But he was looking at it **totally** the wrong way round, because surgical firms don't revolve around him, me, you or any student. They revolve around patients, surgeons, nurses, technicians, anaesthetists, porters, cleaners and countless other staff who keep the operating theatres in action. They all run to their own schedules, and the onus is on us to fit in around that, not to rock up whenever suits us and expect entertaining. He was in fact showing up at the very worst time, when the FY1s and SHOs were at their busiest, and not even sticking around long enough for things to calm down. These juniors were actually keen to teach and we often had great informal sessions in that very same office, but not until 11 or 12, once they had got on top of their most urgent jobs for the day.

One FY1 told me point blank he thought this student was disrespectful for regularly showing up after the ward round – his view was that you come in at 8 a.m. or don't bother. I tend to agree. It was also very inefficient use of time by the student because he did the same thing three or four times a week: given the relaxed rules on attendance, it would have been far better just to pick two days but make the effort to show up early, join the ward round, show some enthusiasm and stick around long enough to get the informal teaching he wanted, then do something else on the other days. Epic fail. Don't be that guy!

### 3.4.4 Clerking 101

I've already mentioned clerking a few times: so what exactly **is** it? Clerking is basically medical-speak for taking a history from a patient and examining them. Some students love clerking and others hate it, but either way it forms a core part of clinical placements so there is no getting away from it. I believe you should learn to love clerking and do it as much as possible, and I'll explain why.

First let's consider the term 'clerking' in more detail as I found it was used inconsistently by different people, which can be very confusing for students at the start of clinical placements. Let's start with this definition from **Segen's Medical Dictionary**[3]:

> "The act of taking a patient's complete history, performing an examination, recording it all in the patient's notes, and writing a problem list and a care plan."

This is what it means at the level of an admitting doctor, such as in A&E, where a full clerking should be a thorough and comprehensive assessment of the patient's symptoms and baseline status when they first get to hospital. It's like a detailed 'checking-in' process, ensuring that all of the patient's problems are catalogued so they can be referred to the right specialty and managed appropriately. Clerking should include an examination of cardio, respiratory, abdominal and neurological systems as a minimum, plus any other relevant examinations. The notes generated from admission clerkings are very important documents, and many hospitals use a structured, standardised template to ensure nothing gets missed. These often include sections for listing which investigations have been ordered and what the provisional diagnosis and management plan are. There are a lot of shorthand symbols which won't make much sense to you at first, so check out **Figure 3.9** for an intro. Geeky Medics also has a great guide to clerking if you want to learn more.[4]

> When you are asked to clerk a patient, briefly clarify what's expected of you before you potter off to the bedside. For example: "Just a history or the complete examination as well?" This will save you a *lot* of trouble when you come to present the case.

**TOP TIP**

At the medical student level, however, the term is used much more loosely. When people ask you to clerk a patient, they can mean anything from 'take a brief history' to 'do the entire history and examination, writing in the notes as you go, then come and present it back to me'. More often than not, I'd say it translates roughly as:

3  https://medical-dictionary.thefreedictionary.com/clerking+in
4  www.geekymedics.com/clearking-101/

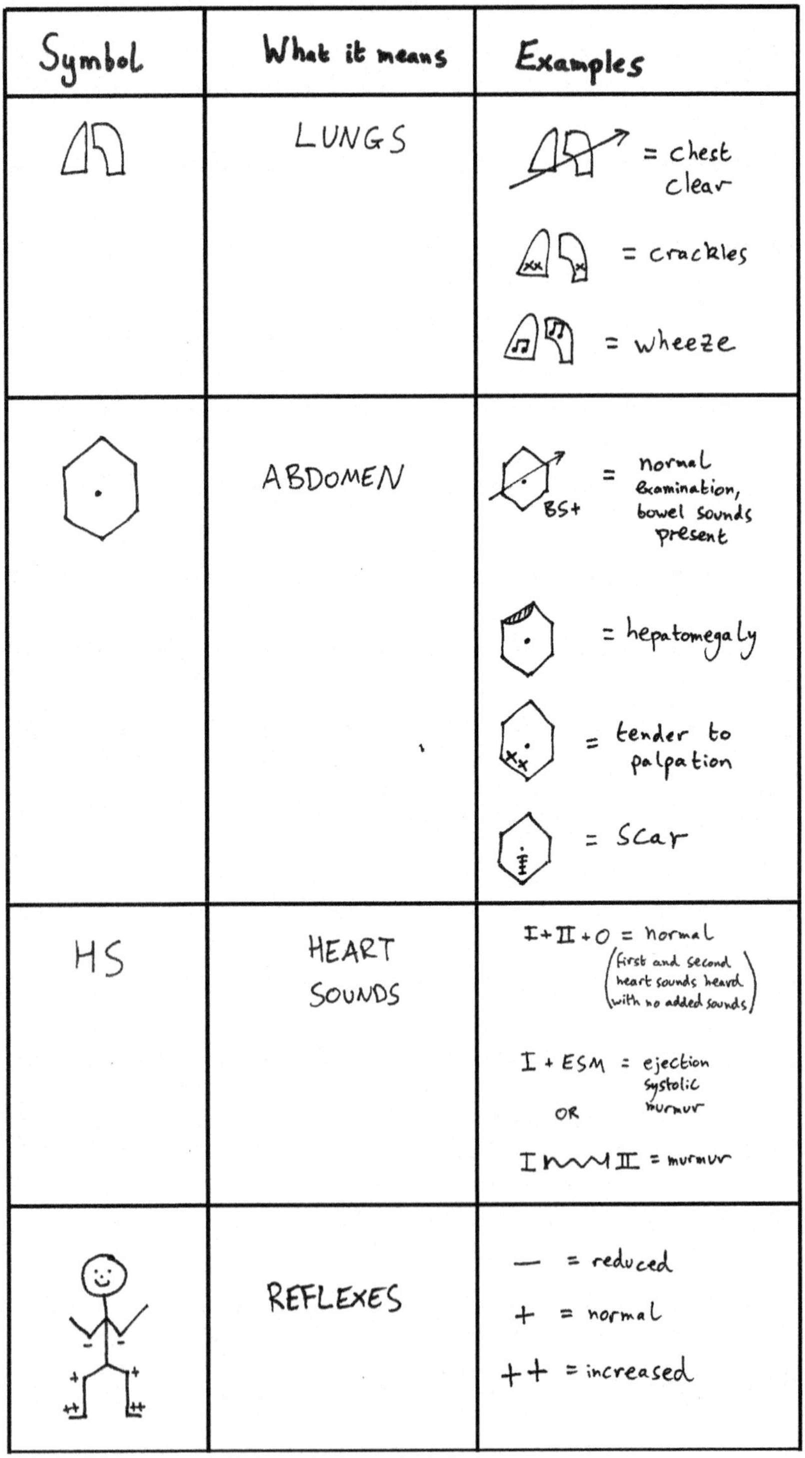

| Symbol | What it means | Examples |
|---|---|---|
| | LUNGS | = chest clear<br><br> = crackles<br><br> = wheeze |
| | ABDOMEN | = normal examination, bowel sounds present<br><br> = hepatomegaly<br><br> = tender to palpation<br><br> = scar |
| HS | HEART SOUNDS | I + II + O = normal (first and second heart sounds heard with no added sounds)<br><br>I + ESM = ejection systolic murmur<br>OR<br>I ∿∿ II = murmur |
| | REFLEXES | — = reduced<br>+ = normal<br>++ = increased |

Figure 3.9: Shorthand symbols commonly used to record examination findings in medical clerkings.

*Take a full history, examine all the major systems but focus your efforts on the bits you think are most relevant, come up with some sort of idea of what is wrong with the patient, then verbally present the case to someone.*

Clerking can be an informal, spontaneous activity, or a formal requirement for passing a placement: for example, you may have to write up a certain number of clerkings, or get a certain number of presentations signed off by a supervisor. **Box 3.7** has some tips to help you get the most out of your clerkings, and hopefully make them more enjoyable in the process.

Clerking can be an amazing learning opportunity yet students often look down on it, for the following reasons:

1. It's hard! You're still learning the communication and examination skills, lack experience, can't recognise patterns yet and have been taught different subjects in a highly compartmentalised way. So to combine everything you've learned into one comprehensive assessment of a real patient can be extremely daunting and time-consuming. And god help you if the patient is a talker – you could be there for hours. Make sure you do a wee first.

2. When presenting back the case, you can easily find yourself on the wrong end of a bollocking, particularly if you don't go into enough detail (**Figure 3.10**). Or the reverse: you present your findings in immense detail and get laughed off the ward for wasting your time on completely irrelevant examinations. "I was unable to complete my full examination because the patient fell asleep" is probably a bad thing to be saying (yup, I've been there).

3. It feels like a thankless task: people will happily list all the things you missed, reel off 20 ways your presentation could be improved and tell you at length why your diagnosis makes no sense. It is much less common that they will praise you for a good clerking.

4. It feels like a 'default' activity to give medical students when there's nothing better to do. You're not stupid, you can tell what's just gone down: "Uh oh the medical students are here … erm … what we gonna do with them? Ermmmmmmmmm … can we ask them to go and get us coffees? Probably not. Do that lumbar puncture we've been putting off? Not a chance. Ooooh I know! Go and clerk the geezer in bed ten! Phew … that got rid of them for a while …"

5. You have to actually talk to real patients. It's surprising how many medical students dread doing this.

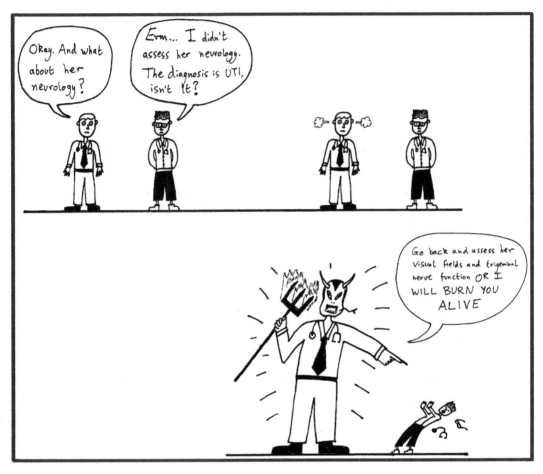

**Figure 3.10: You can easily find yourself on the wrong end of a grilling if you don't go into enough detail when clerking and presenting a patient.** Avoid this fate by clarifying what's expected of you up front.

There is substance to those concerns, I hear you loud and clear. But here are my counterarguments, in defence of clerking:

1. Yes it's hard, but this is how we learn! Clerking gives you an opportunity to practise, try new things and hone your skills in a safe space, just you and the patient, free from the pressure of an OSCE or an overbearing consultant. You can breezily tell the registrar "Heart sounds were normal", omitting the fact that you spent five minutes listening with your stethoscope the wrong way round before frantically telling the nearest nurse that the patient was clinically dead. Practising will make you slicker, more confident and less prone to making such clangers. Clerking is also a great way to build up your pattern recognition.

**Top tips for getting the most out of clerking patients**

Box 3.7

- Use patients as a hook to learn about a topic. Try to remember their faces, their voices, their social situations and their stories. Understand what symptoms they've been experiencing and how the disease has impacted their lives. If you're anything like me, you'll find it much easier to remember information that has a human face to it.
- Clerk in pairs to begin with. This makes it quicker and easier as you can divide up the tasks, e.g. one of you can examine while the other takes the history. You can also give each other moral support, provide friendly feedback and bounce ideas around before giving your presentation.
- Appreciate that patients are often delighted to talk to a medical student. It might be no big deal to you, but to them you're potentially the first staff member who has actually pulled up a chair and properly listened to what they have to say. Being in hospital can be lonely, boring and frightening, and you can do the world of good by providing a friendly, smiling face who doesn't rush off after two minutes.
- Keep track of patients you have clerked. Take an interest in how their case unfolds and pop over to say hi whenever you pass their bed. It's much more enjoyable getting to know one patient properly than trying to get your head around 30 you've never met.
- Present cases to your seniors as much as possible. This is a core skill, which we will talk about in more detail in the next chapter (*Section 4.5.2*). But for now just take every opportunity to practise presenting, get feedback and learn from it, even if the learning curve feels very steep to begin with. This will stand you in excellent stead later on if you can overcome your initial reservations and throw yourself into this early on.
- Clerk in the dark. Not literally – that would be weird – but try to approach a patient *without* knowing their diagnosis and what investigations and management they have already received, as you can learn a lot more this way. Ask the patient at the beginning not to reveal this to you. Then once you have completed your history and examination, challenge yourself to come up with a thorough list of differentials and further investigations.

**2.** It's not just medical students whose patient presentations get savaged: I have seen senior registrars get publicly torn to shreds by consultants who really should know better, and have even witnessed consultants yelling at each other. It's not right but it does happen, and you can hopefully avoid this fate by improving your presentations through practice and experience. And the good news is, as a med student no one actually expects very much of you, so you can really wow people once you get the hang of it.

3. Negative feedback might be hard to take but it can still be extremely useful. Swallow your pride, write everything down in your notebook and try to improve for next time. And make a mental note to be a nice person who gives positive feedback when students present their clerkings to you in future!

4. The flip side to being a 'default' activity is that it also serves as a universally accepted currency for teaching. You can walk onto any ward in any NHS hospital, introduce yourself and ask the doctors, "Have you got any interesting patients for me to clerk?" They will immediately understand what you are asking, make some suggestions and hopefully invite you to present the patient back to them later. This gives you an 'in', helping you forge that all-important human connection with ward doctors and hopefully securing yourself some informal teaching in the process. Much better than awkwardly lingering at the entrance to the doctors' office hoping someone will talk to you.

5. It's natural to feel nervous and awkward when you first begin talking to real patients, but this should start to wear off with practice. If you really feel you are struggling with it then don't just bury your head in the sand and hope the problem will go away because it won't: speaking to patients is an absolutely core part of the career you've chosen (unless you become a pathologist or radiologist). Get help and advice from a senior or a tutor, and encourage yourself to keep practising until it starts to feel easier.

## 3.4.5 Common things are common

"Common things are common" is a saying that gets bandied around *a lot* at medical school. I initially found it one of the stupidest, most annoying phrases I'd ever heard, because it seemed patronising, self-evident, and completely unhelpful. And when you're first taught it in the cold, detached light of a lecture theatre, I think that reaction is probably fair. I put it out of my mind and hoped no one would mention it to me ever again.

On clinical placements, however, this phrase starts to gradually make sense. And eventually I came to find it very useful and important – hence I want you to appreciate it too (you may have heard it phrased differently: see *Box 3.8*). Essentially it's something to remind yourself *any time* you

**Alternative versions of "common things are common"**

You'll probably hear all of these on placements: use whichever floats your boat, provided it helps you remember the concept.
- "The simplest explanation is usually correct" (Occam's razor)
- "When you hear hoofbeats, think of horses not zebras"
- "If it looks like a duck, swims like a duck, and quacks like a duck, then it probably is a duck"

are clerking or presenting a patient, or formulating a list of differential diagnoses. Because yes, the concept is self-explanatory, but somehow in the heat of the moment **we forget it over and over again**. Particularly as medical students, we tend to get overexcited about rare and obscure diagnoses and overlook the far more obvious explanation. At your stage of training, and even mine, this is a bad strategy which can make us look silly and potentially lose us marks.

So what are you to do? Essentially any time you are considering what's wrong with a patient, state the most common of the potential diagnoses first. More often than not it will be right, and you will demonstrate to your listener that you understand basic logic, statistics and reasoning. Causes of small bowel obstruction? Adhesions and hernias, not Mirizzi's syndrome or gallstone ileus. Causes of pancreatitis? Gallstones and alcohol, not mumps and scorpion stings.[5] Patient presenting with fever, tachycardia and confusion? Sepsis, not neuroleptic fricking malignant syndrome.

I'm not saying you can't show off by knowing the obscure stuff – but leave it until last and add caveats making clear you understand that it is rare and therefore less likely. Believe me, I've learned this the hard way: you go from feeling very clever to very stupid in a matter of seconds, and you are very rarely correct! You'll be expected to know every rare diagnosis under the sun when you're a registrar or consultant, but until then it's a much better strategy to try to play it safe.

> When presenting differential diagnoses, always go with the most common and likely explanations first. Open with the rare and obscure ones and one in 100 times you're a genius, but 99 you're a plonker.

---

5 This is where mnemonics like I GET SMASHED (*Section 2.4.7*) can inadvertently cause you grief. Use them to help you remember everything, but try to rearrange them into a more sensible order before presenting out loud so you don't look silly!

## 3.4.6 Time management on clinical placements

For most students on clinical placements, the single biggest challenge in terms of time management is when to attend and when to skive off. You'll probably have a few compulsory hours per week of formal teaching, and as a rule I would suggest you attend all of these because you will learn a lot from these sessions, particularly 'bedside teaching' which focuses on your history taking and examination skills (**Section 3.6.1**). Also, they are usually delivered by actual doctors who are taking time out of their busy days to teach you, and it creates a very bad impression to not attend! Try to read up in advance so you can engage with the topic and get the most out of it.

> **TOP TIP**
>
> Always attend timetabled teaching sessions on placement, particularly those designated as 'bedside teaching'. These give you invaluable practice at taking histories and examining real patients, with useful feedback which you can use in your OSCEs.

But compulsory sessions aside, there will also be loads of unstructured time, usually afternoons, where your timetable simply says 'attend ward' or 'clerking'. Essentially these sessions are putting the ball in your court as to how to spend your time.

I think the decision whether to stay or go during these periods is very simple: it comes entirely down to whether you are learning anything (**Figure 3.11**). You might have pegged me as a massive nerd who spent every last minute on the ward but that's really not the case: my approach was to show up bright and early most mornings, try to extract the most out of the learning opportunities on offer then head off as soon I felt things drying up. I encourage you to do the same.

**Try your best to engineer teaching opportunities for yourself using all the tactics we have discussed, but if it ain't happening, it ain't happening. Don't just hang around all afternoon twiddling your thumbs and getting ignored!**

Remember you are a **student**, not a paid employee (in fact, you are paying to be there!): your obligation is to yourself and your studies, not to slavishly following a generic timetable. You also have a golden window to consolidate your new-found knowledge while it is still fresh in your mind, so go to the library, a coffee shop, wherever, and spend an hour or two looking back over your notes, reading up and doing a few practice questions

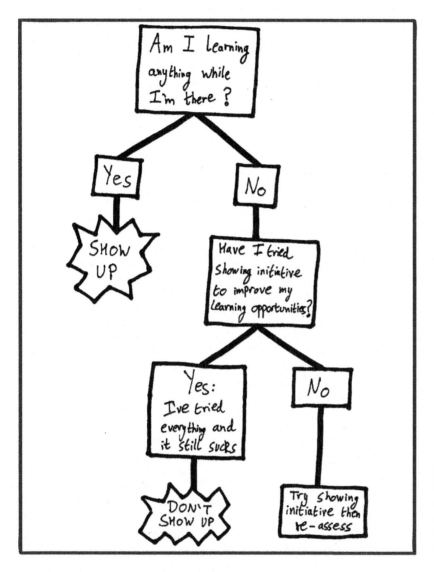

**Figure 3.11: Should I bother showing up for unstructured time on clinical placements?** Use this simple decision tree to help you decide.

before you go home. This is time excellently spent and an important way to consolidate your learning from wards, clinics and theatres.

Another time management tip is that in general, it is always a better strategy to 'front-load' a clinical placement, i.e. to start enthusiastic then ease off later on, rather than the other way around. Being new to a department provides a great opportunity to introduce yourself, establish connections, allow people to make positive first impressions of you, get to know the place, ask dumb questions with impunity and establish the interesting patients and the high-yield topics. By immersing yourself over the first couple of weeks, you can extract a lot from a placement then confidently make decisions about how best to spend your time for the rest of it.

Pissing around for the first few weeks, on the other hand, means you are missing these opportunities, pressurising yourself to cram your learning into a shorter space of time, playing catch-up with the other students and jeopardising your sign-off. This is a remarkably common pitfall! I was once on placement with a student who failed to show up for the very first session on the very first Monday morning – a meet and greet with the consultant who would be supervising us for the next five weeks – without sending any excuse or apologies. The consultant was deeply unimpressed, made a point of finding out the student's name and was heavily on their case for the rest of the placement. Flagging yourself up as a slacker on day one is an absolutely terrible strategy!

> **TOP TIP**
>
> On clinical placements, 'front-load' by going hard for the first couple of weeks. Then you can decide whether or not to ease off for the rest of it, based on how good the placement is and how much you are learning. Doing it the opposite way around – starting slack then trying to lean in towards the end – really doesn't work as well.

It is also very important to carefully check your university's requirements on attendance levels and sign-off, as you really don't want to fail a placement for poor attendance. Your university will probably consider it a professionalism issue, which will do you no favours to have on your record. I would suggest leaving yourself some leeway: if minimum attendance is 80%, and you are targeting this exact level throughout your placement, you are very vulnerable should you get sick or have some other crisis in the last week which necessitates a few days off. Better to give yourself a cushion and expect the unexpected.

At my med school, I heard about a low-attending student who pulled a sickie towards the end of a placement, thinking they were safe to take one day off without falling below the minimum attendance level. But they made the mistake of saying they had a 'stomach bug': this allowed the consultant, who knew full well the student was taking the piss, to call them out by pointing out the hospital policy stating that staff with diarrhoea and vomiting had to take at least three days off. The student couldn't very well argue with this! But three days off pushed them under the attendance line, causing them to fail the placement and, apparently, the year. I can't entirely vouch for the veracity of this story but knowing the consultant involved, it is 100% plausible!

> **TOP TIP**
>
> Don't sail too close to the wind with attendance on clinical placements. Give yourself plenty of leeway in case you get genuinely ill or something unexpected happens which requires you to take time off.

Finally, make sure you put in enough face time with the specific person who is due to sign you off, making an effort to attend their clinics, ask questions and so on. You don't want to hand them your sign-off sheet on the last day, only for them to say "Sorry but I've never seen you before in my life". These are intelligent people – they will notice if you suddenly start attending every day in the final week of a long placement, having never shown your face before! And they might even ask the junior doctors or nurses whether you've actually spent any time on the wards, which is where showing your face during those unstructured afternoons can come in extremely handy.

## 3.4.7  The pros and cons of FY1s

At the time of writing I'm an FY1 (not, as one of my non-medic friends thought my badge said, an 'FYI doctor'). I graduated medical school just nine months ago, so it all still feels very fresh in my mind. Hence when medical students come to my wards I feel like I can relate to them, because I remember all too well that odd mixture of excitement, intrigue, fear, boredom and uselessness on clinical placements. So I make an effort to talk to them, teach them and make them feel included as best as I can.

**FY1s want to help you, because we were you not so long ago.**

For these reasons, you will find that you naturally gravitate towards FY1s and FY2s on clinical placements and probably spend more time with them than with other seniority grades. This is fantastic – you are most welcome to join us – but I do want to make you aware of our strengths and limitations. In **Table 3.4** we'll consider, from the medical student perspective, some of the pros and cons of FY1s compared to more senior doctors such as registrars and consultants. Senior house officers (SHOs) lie somewhere in the middle: this term is usually applied to doctors from the start of FY2 up to the end of their second year of specialty training. Registrars are further along a specialty training pathway: usually somewhere between their third and eighth year, depending on the specialty.

By arming yourself with this knowledge you can hopefully hit the ground running on clinical placements by playing to our strengths and weaknesses. Ask me to listen to your case presentation or talk you through routine blood tests; don't ask me why certain guidelines have been

**Table 3.4: The pros and cons of FY1s compared to more senior doctors.** These are worth bearing in mind as you navigate clinical placements for the first time. Note that FY1s change placements every four months and don't get much choice over which placements they do.

| | Pros | Cons |
|---|---|---|
| **FY1s** | • Closer to you in age and life stage, easier to relate to <br><br> • Can offer pointers on surviving medical school, Foundation Programme applications, etc. <br><br> • Knowledge calibration: they'll know which topics you do and don't need to know for finals <br><br> • Consistently accessible: they are usually on the ward day in day out, 9–5 <br><br> • Knowledgeable about basic procedures, prescribing, documentation, specific patients and day-to-day life on the wards <br><br> • Great for providing informal teaching later in the day <br><br> • They're doing what you will be doing when you graduate | • Inexperienced <br><br> • Not necessarily knowledgeable or passionate about the specialty they're currently working in <br><br> • Won't be able to answer lots of academic-type questions, or may give wrong answers <br><br> • Tend to be busiest and most stressed early in the day, particularly during ward rounds <br><br> • Often powerless to engage with you on ward rounds, even if they want to <br><br> • Spend lots of their time on boring tasks such as paperwork, which are unhelpful to you |
| **Registrars and consultants** | • Experienced <br><br> • Sometimes inspirational <br><br> • Knowledgeable and passionate about their specialty, usually up to date, able to answer all your questions <br><br> • Provide formal teaching <br><br> • Lead ward rounds and clinics, so if they want to take things slowly and get you involved, that's their prerogative <br><br> • Take the lead in surgery and for advanced medical procedures such as chest drain insertions, which are great to observe <br><br> • May be directly involved with your exams and OSCEs <br><br> • Responsible for your sign-off | • Can't remember what it's like to be a medical student <br><br> • Sometimes intimidating and unapproachable <br><br> • Not always interested in teaching: if they set the tone for a rapid, non-teaching ward round or clinic, you're stuffed <br><br> • Older consultants' knowledge and style can be outdated <br><br> • Not always around, particularly in afternoons <br><br> • Their jobs are far removed from what you will be doing once you graduate <br><br> • Won't help you with basic procedures such as taking blood |

changed or what I think about the latest clinical trial in the **New England Journal of Medicine**. Put those questions to the consultant, but don't ask them to supervise you inserting a cannula. Ultimately you will benefit from getting different types of teaching from all of the seniority grades, so tailor your requests appropriately and we will usually be happy to help!

### 3.4.8 Answering questions

A massive part of clinical placements is being asked questions, questions and more questions. And not so much "Where did you get those awesome shoes?" or "So … what are your thoughts on Brexit?", but more: "What are the potential complications of this surgery?", "What can you tell me about the management of osteoarthritis?" and "What are the causes of diarrhoea?". Questioning, aka grilling, is a completely accepted form of teaching in the medical profession the world over, so I'm afraid you'll need to get used to it!

> You will be asked a *lot* of questions on placements as a way to assess your knowledge, particularly by consultants. Developing clear and logical structures to your answers will help you out enormously.

**KEY POINT**

The thing no one tells you is that it's not just about answering questions **correctly**, but it's also about how you **structure** your answers. In fact having a good structure can be almost as important as having the knowledge, because it allows you to save face and salvage some credit even when you get the answer wrong. The other great thing about a well-structured answer is that it buys you more thinking time while you retrieve the information from the dusty recesses of your brain, and prompts you to cover bases you might otherwise forget.

This is a skill that takes a lot of discipline and patience to master, so it's good to start early and get plenty of practice. The first thing to do whenever you are asked a broad, open-ended question on placement is to resist the urge to blurt out an answer immediately; instead pause, take a deep breath and start thinking about your structure. Just by doing this simple step you are getting yourself off on the right foot. And don't worry about looking slow: it is completely acceptable to have some thinking time, and most doctors would prefer you thought about your answer carefully than said the first thing that came into your mind.

> Any time you are asked a clinical question on placement, pause, take a deep breath and consider how to structure your answer. This will get you more credit than blurting out the first thing that comes into your head.

**TOP TIP**

There are loads of different structures you can use to answer questions, depending on the situation (**Box 3.9**). Let's start by looking at the examples above, all of which I have been asked in my time:

*Q: What are the potential complications of this surgery?*

This is a tried-and-tested classic, which any surgeon can ask about any procedure. A great structure to use here is to divide your answer into immediate, short- and long-term complications. Let's say we're talking about a thyroidectomy. If you paid attention in anatomy you probably want to shout out "RECURRENT LARYNGEAL NERVE INJURY!!!" at the top of your voice and be super-pleased with yourself. Resist! Pause, take a deep breath, and:

*A: The potential complications of a thyroidectomy can be divided into immediate, short- and long-term. In the immediate term, during surgery, there are risks of bleeding and injury to the recurrent laryngeal nerve or parathyroid glands. In the short term, postoperative risks include wound infection, seroma formation, airway obstruction and acute hypocalcaemia. The main long-term complication is chronic hypocalcaemia.*

This is a very logical way to answer this question and I assure you surgeons will dig it, even if you didn't remember all the bits of information. Another great thing about this particular structure is that you can include bleeding and infection as complications of **absolutely any** surgical procedure, so

**Box 3.9**

**Some tried-and-tested ways to structure your answers when being grilled on clinical placements:**

*Q: What are the complications of ...*

A: Immediate vs. short-term vs. long-term
    Most serious to least serious
    Most common to least common

*Q: What is the management of ...*

A: Conservative vs. medical vs. surgical
    First line vs. second line vs. third line

*Q: What are the causes of ...*

A: Surgical sieve, e.g. VITAMIN CDEF (*Section 2.6.6*)

that's two freebies which you might have overlooked if you'd jumped straight to a specific complication. Other ways to answer this question would be to go from the most serious to the least serious, or from the most common to the least common. Surgeons also like these answers because they are very pragmatic, suggesting that you have considered how these complications actually play out in the real world. These are all valid structures so just go with whichever you prefer and feel you can pull off in the moment.

Let's move onto the second example:

*Q: What can you tell me about the management of osteoarthritis?*

Another classic. You can interchange 'osteoarthritis' with virtually any disease and you'll find a consultant somewhere who likes to ask this of their medical students. A very handy and widely accepted structure for this type of question is to split your answer into conservative, medical and surgical approaches, as follows:

*A: The management of osteoarthritis can be divided into conservative, medical and surgical approaches. Conservative measures include weight loss, physiotherapy, stretches and strengthening exercises. Medical management includes analgesia such as paracetamol and NSAIDs, steroid tablets and injections. Surgical measures include joint repair and replacement.*

I love this structure for two main reasons. First, it is pragmatic because this is the order in which treatments are likely to be tried in the real world. You will look silly if you blurt out 'hip replacement' as your opening answer because surgery is reserved as a last-line option for when everything else has failed: if GPs referred every patient for surgery without trying the other things first then the entire world's orthopaedic system would grind to a halt overnight. Secondly, this structure forces you to cover the conservative approaches, which most students forget to mention because they're not as cool or sexy as drugs and surgery. So you'll look good if you spell these out first.

And the third example:

*Q: What are the causes of diarrhoea?*

A consultant gastroenterologist asked me this in my penultimate year while I was observing her perform a colonoscopy. It is an unbelievably broad question: there must be hundreds of different causes of diarrhoea! Did she really want me to list them all?? Fortunately she gave me some thinking time (while casually feeding the probe deeper into the patient's arse) so I was able to pick my structure carefully. I opted for the surgical sieve outlined in **Section 2.6.6**, answering something like:

*A: There are lots of causes of diarrhoea, including infective, inflammatory, autoimmune, iatrogenic and neoplastic causes…*

This episode stands out in my mind because the consultant actually stopped me at this point and said "Well done" for setting my answer out clearly. She explained that she asks students this question a lot, precisely **because** it is so broad, and what she really wants to see is whether they can break it down into a coherent structure. Tick boom! From there, with the battle already won, I felt much more comfortable going into specifics:

*Infective causes include bacterial infections such as* E. coli, C. difficile *and cholera, viruses such as norovirus, and parasitic infections such as* Giardia. *Inflammatory causes include Crohn's disease and ulcerative colitis. Autoimmune causes include coeliac disease. Iatrogenic causes include laxative abuse and side-effects of medications such as metformin. Neoplastic causes include bowel cancer. And so on…*

I'm grateful to this consultant for her honesty in confirming that this hidden agenda often underlies the questions they ask us! I'm not sure anyone else explicitly admitted this during my entire time at medical school. Unfortunately, however, it's rare that a consultant actually praises you for the structure of your answer. They take it for granted that you will answer with a clear structure and don't acknowledge it when you do, but then criticise you when you don't. I think this is extremely unfair! But all you can do is keep practising until a good structure becomes second nature, then silently high five yourself when you do it well.

There are probably infinite ways you can structure answers, but **Table 3.5** has a few more options, with examples. Whichever structure you pick, make sure it allows you to cover the most important, common and simple things. Some consultants will be delighted to discuss obscure minutiae with you, but most would rather see that you are more focused on everyday topics. Jumping straight to the small print can also make it look like you are showing off, which is a sure-fire way to make yourself unpopular with both the consultant and your peers!

**KEY POINT**

A word of caution: not *all* questions give you options for structuring your answer. Some have specific structures which you are widely expected to use. For example, the causes of acute kidney injury should be divided into pre-renal, intrinsic renal and post-renal, the causes of jaundice into pre-hepatic, hepatic and post-hepatic, and the causes of pleural effusions into transudates and exudates. Don't worry about these for now: you will be taught them when the time is right!

One final point to consider when answering questions on placements. You might have noticed that I have repeatedly used the words 'includes' and 'such as' in my answers. This is a deliberate strategy which has evolved in response to a great many slap-downs. The point is to be broad rather than specific – to keep your options open and avoid sounding too definitive. For example, by saying "Autoimmune causes of diarrhoea **include** coeliac disease" you are allowing for the fact that there might be loads of other autoimmune causes which you can't remember right now. If you had said "The only autoimmune cause of diarrhoea is coeliac disease" then you have revealed your ignorance about other causes, when you could easily have brushed this under the carpet and got away with it! Another beautiful little phrase to start using is 'would consider'. This comes in super-handy when asked how you would manage a particular patient or condition; for example, "I would consider steroid injections" is a better answer than "I would give a steroid injection" because it keeps your options open and shows that you appreciate not every patient will be suitable for a steroid injection. I realise this might sound pernickety but trust me, you'll have

**Table 3.5: More examples of ways to structure your answers to questions on clinical placements.** Note that there are often lots of different options for answering the same question. You just need to pick one and go with it!

| Structure | Example question | Example answer |
|---|---|---|
| First line vs. second line vs. third line | What is the management of supraventricular tachycardia in a haemodynamically stable patient? | First-line management involves vagal manoeuvres such as carotid sinus massage; if that is unsuccessful, progress to IV adenosine as second line, followed by a calcium channel blocker or beta blocker as third line |
| Group by body system (a variant of the surgical sieve) | What might be causing this patient's shortness of breath? | Respiratory causes include asthma and COPD, cardiac causes include heart failure, haematological causes include anaemia, and so on |
| Anatomical, e.g. medial vs. lateral | What are the causes of neck lumps? | Midline lumps include goitres and thyroglossal cysts; lateral lumps include lymph nodes, aneurysms and lipomas |
| From inside the vessel to outside | What are the causes of bowel obstruction? | Intraluminal causes include foreign bodies and faecal impaction; luminal causes include colorectal cancers and strictures; extraluminal causes include volvulus, hernias and adhesions |
| Local vs. distant | What are the complications of lung cancer? | Local effects include pain, shortness of breath, haemoptysis and pleural effusions; distant effects include metastasis and paraneoplastic syndromes such as SIADH |

> **Avoid being too specific in your answers: keep them broad by using handy phrases like "I would *consider*" or "causes *include*". This makes you look well clever by showing off the stuff you know while disguising the stuff you don't.**

consultants eating out of the palm of your hand in no time! Or just preferentially bollocking someone else, which is good too.

### 3.4.9 Procedures/DOPs

As if ward rounds, clinics, theatres, clerkings and regular grillings weren't enough, clinical placements also provide your first opportunity to start doing practical procedures on actual live human beings. By which I mean taking blood, inserting cannulas and nasogastric tubes, putting catheters into bladders and much, much more. If you're really super-lucky, you might even get to put your finger up someone else's bottom. How many of your friends get to do *that* at work, eh?

> **No matter how much you practise on those weird rubber arms in clinical skills teaching, nothing can truly prepare you for the experience of getting blood out of a real, living human being and into a little plastic bottle.**

Now then. Procedures are another of those things that seem totally, utterly terrifying when you start medical school. I remember how nervous I was the first time I actually punctured someone else's skin with a needle: I felt like I was committing a heinous crime for which I ought to be arrested.

We'll look at some specific tips for performing procedures in the next chapter (**Section 4.5.6**), but there are a few things you need to know right away. First: you will fail at procedures. Over and over again. Put your perfectionist, OCD tendencies aside and just accept this fact! No one was born with mad cannulation skills – they learned the hard way through trial, error and practice, practice, practice. You will learn too, so I implore you not to be hard on yourself when you inevitably struggle to begin with. And certainly do not compare yourself to the registrar, nurse or phlebotomist who swans in and makes everything look ridiculously easy. They've been jabbing people since you were in nappies, so give yourself a break! Be polite and professional, try it up to three times if the patient is happy for you to do so, then graciously accept defeat and get someone more senior to do it.

Procedures such as venepuncture take a lot of practice and you won't always be successful. Just keep working on it and don't be hard on yourself when it doesn't work out.

**KEY POINT**

This brings me on to my second point: when it comes to procedures, there simply is no substitute for practice. I wish I could give you a shortcut, or a magic trick to make everything easier, but the fact is you just need to don those gloves and get stuck in whenever possible. Be sure to observe a couple of times before doing anything yourself, and get someone to supervise your initial attempts at a new skill. Get their feedback and learn from it. But don't hide behind your inexperience as a medical student by passing up opportunities – I know I did this on occasions and I regret it. Challenge yourself to do as many as you can to get over the jitters and eventually you will start to get the hang of it. In the short term, this will help you create a good impression on your placements and to look slick and polished when procedures come up in your OSCEs. And in the longer term you're ensuring you start work as a doctor with the skills required to do your job. Trust me, when you're an FY1 experiencing the horror of weekend ward cover, there will be nowhere to hide when someone needs to be bled, cannulated or catheterised.

Force yourself to do as many procedures as possible until you get comfortable and competent. Don't use inexperience as an excuse to pass up opportunities.

**TOP TIP**

I'm referring here to opportunities which present themselves spontaneously during placements. But you will probably also have a certain number of compulsory procedures to do in order to pass the block, usually called DOPs (directly observed procedures). Here, someone observes you perform a skill and then signs something to state that you have done it.

DOPs can seem like a complete pain in the rectum but deep down you'll realise they are a good thing because they drag you out of your comfort zone and force you to at least attempt all the core procedures. The other great thing about them is that they'll give you an 'in' to establish connections with doctors on your team – we have to do DOPs throughout our careers so everyone is very understanding about your need to get them signed off. Use this to start a conversation by explaining nice and early that you need to get DOPs done, and asking when would be a good time for someone to supervise you and give you some pointers. Hopefully they'll make some time for you and maybe even throw in a bit of informal teaching. Target your requests to kind, calm, patient people who will be sympathetic if you mess it up! They've almost certainly been there themselves. And check whether you can get your DOPs signed off by nurses: often they are highly skilled at procedures such as cannulation and you can learn absolutely loads from them.

**TOP TIP**

> Get your mandatory DOPs signed off as early as possible so you can relax and forget about them.

Make sure you are organised and proactive and get your DOPs done and signed off as early as possible. You can't magically order up procedures according to your own schedule (I know, patients are so selfish, right?), so you need to grab the opportunities when they present themselves.

**It is remarkably common to find medical students running around the hospital on the last day of the last term asking: "Anyone need an arterial blood gas done?" This is a disastrous strategy in the run-up to exams, when the last thing you need is added stress. Don't put yourself in that position!**

## 3.4.10 Electronic vs. paper records

One of the challenges facing you as a medical student now is that you are living through the NHS's changeover from paper to electronic records. As a student, I had placements on wards which were mostly paper-based, others which were fully computerised, and others which were anywhere in between. And as an FY1 I've had to live through the turmoil of my hospital switching from paper to electronic, and will likely have to do it all over again at a different hospital in FY2. Sigh.

You probably haven't thought about this much, but the introduction of electronic records has a huge impact on you as a student on clinical placements. And despite the many obvious advantages of electronic records, unfortunately for medical students I'd say on balance they're a negative development. Mainly because they dramatically reduce your access to patient information: without a smartcard and all the right electronic permissions you can't read the documentation, check blood test results or look at scans by yourself (*Figure 3.12*). This makes it almost impossible to figure out what's going on from a clinical perspective. Placements absolutely suck when you can't find out the most basic information about patients. On paper-based wards, by contrast, you are free to pick up the

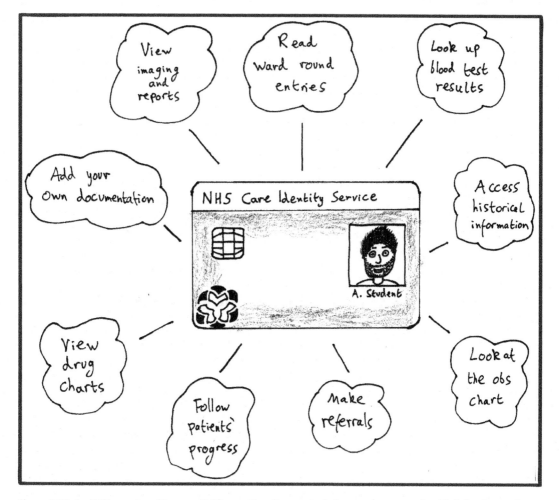

**Figure 3.12: An NHS smartcard is essential for making the most of placements on wards with fully electronic documentation.** Without one, you will struggle to learn even the most basic information about the patients.

patient's folder whenever no one else is using it and digest this information at your own pace (assuming of course that you respect confidentiality and follow any rules or guidance your medical school has around accessing patient records).

In reality, this means that on computer-based wards you are often reduced to looking over someone's shoulder while they type on ward rounds, or to asking whether you can look up a few things on their login. This is very unsatisfactory and can make you feel like a nuisance for always asking.

The solution is to push **hard** to get yourself the electronic access that you need. Your medical school should be routinely providing students with a smartcard and some level of read-only access to patient records. Getting this set up, in my experience, can be an utterly painful process involving multiple calls to IT and visits to various back offices in parts of the hospital you never even knew existed. But take a deep breath and persevere, because your learning experience will be vastly improved if you can get it sorted. And if your medical school isn't providing this access, then ask them why not and push to get the situation changed. Don't take no for an answer on this: there really isn't a lot of point in having placements where students can't look up the most basic clinical information!

**KEY POINT**

The introduction of electronic health records can have a negative impact on your learning experience by reducing your access to patient information. Avoid this by getting set up as early as possible with a smartcard and the right permissions. This can be tricky but persevere!

## 3.4.11  How 'good' is this placement?

You've probably noticed that medical schools love getting feedback from students nowadays. If yours is anything like mine, they probably just emailed you a survey in the time it took you to read this sentence. Clinical placements are no exception: they will want to hear all about how it went and how much support and teaching you got.

This raises a very important but neglected question: how do you actually decide whether a clinical placement is any good? Sure, there are some straightforward factual elements such as whether formal teaching took place as scheduled and covered the topics it was supposed to, but by and large the experience is highly subjective. What one student loves, another might hate, and vice versa. Some want to be constantly challenged; others are happiest when left entirely to their own devices. Chances are, you'll decide fairly quickly whether or not you are enjoying a placement, but it'll be based more on your vague gut feelings than any sort of objective measure.

To fill this void, I'd like to introduce you to a (highly scientific) graph I formulated during my years at medical school, which provides a helpful way to think about clinical placements. Any placement can be plotted simply as a function of educational value versus day-to-day enjoyability, as shown in *Figure 3.13*.

Now let's divide the graph into different zones, as per *Figure 3.14*, which we shall name as follows:

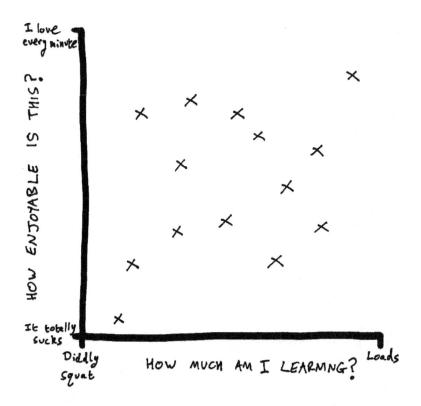

I love every minute

?.

HOW ENJOYABLE IS THIS

It totally sucks

Diddly squat

HOW MUCH AM I LEARNING?

Loads

Figure 3.13: How 'good' is your clinical placement? Plot it on this graph to find out.

Figure 3.13: How 'good' is your clinical placement? Plot it on this graph to find out.

**A = the Comfort Zone. High enjoyability, low learning.** This placement is super-relaxed. Everyone is lovely, you come and go as you please, there's a free coffee machine and unlimited supply of biscuits. But unfortunately no one is teaching you anything. The juniors don't see it as their responsibility, the consultants are never around, the nurses are too busy, there's no turnover of patients and you've already clerked them all. Ah well, better just head off home. After stuffing your pockets with custard creams.

**B = Living the Dream. High enjoyability, high learning.** All the perks above **and** a fantastic learning environment. You're getting bedside teaching and tutorials, doing loads of procedures and feel like a true part of the team. Your notebook is full of learning points from interesting patients you've met who all suffer from high-yield diseases and exclusively take medications which you need to know about for finals. Bring on the exams, because you're gonna ace them.

**C = the Temple of Doom. Low enjoyability, low learning.** This placement has nothing going for it. At best, everyone ignores you; at worst they shout at you and make you feel like an asshole just for showing up. Staff morale is through the floor, you're discouraged from interacting with

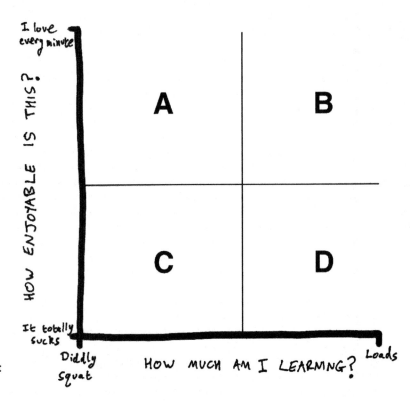

Figure 3.14: Once you've plotted your placement, consider which of these zones it falls into.

patients, the water cooler is broken and, worst of all, you can't even get 4G phone reception. By day three, you're seriously debating whether to even bother showing up.

**D = Baptism by Fire. Low enjoyability, high learning.** This placement evokes mixed feelings. The ward is hot and crowded, students are expected in at the crack of dawn, the consultant sets you daily homework and grills you relentlessly on a head-spinning array of topics: ECGs on Monday, pyramidal versus extrapyramidal side-effects on Tuesday, obscure fish toxins and ancient Greek on Wednesday. You get told off for not putting your gloves and apron on fast enough, for absent-mindedly putting your pen in your mouth, for having facial hair and for standing in the wrong place. But you reflect at the end of week one and realise you have learned an absolutely huge amount. Mostly through a combination of fear and adrenaline, but learned it nonetheless.

You'll experience most of these placements in some form or another throughout medical school, and possibly even the whole range. Type B is perfection – this is what we all want but don't always get, so if you are lucky enough to find yourself on such a placement be sure to recognise your good fortune and ensure you make the most of it! Type C is so bad you should report it to your medical school and try to get moved somewhere else. Let's set both of these aside and focus on A and D.

My impression is that most students, if forced to choose, would pick type A over D – prioritising convenience and comfort over the learning experience. I would argue that to be a top student, you should turn this on its head and embrace type D, by throwing yourself into challenging placements and extracting the most out of them.

**This is where a thick skin becomes an asset, because the discomfort is only temporary, whereas the learning is permanent. It's all about tolerating short-term pain for long-term gain.**

My first-ever clinical placement was a type D and the description above is all true. The lead consultant was notorious for grilling medical students: just saying his name was akin to mentioning Voldemort in the corridors of Hogwarts. There were six of us students on the placement and I found it interesting to observe the different coping strategies. The others mostly chose a middle ground of showing up to just enough of the consultant's ward rounds that he would recognise their faces and sign them off, but arranging to attend clinics or other activities most mornings so they would have a good excuse to avoid his grillings. Some just skived wherever possible. Me, I swallowed my pride and showed up every morning, often finding myself the only medical student on the receiving end of a lengthy interrogation with my back to the wall in a narrow corridor. My sweat patches got so extreme I had to upgrade to a medicated antiperspirant at the end of my first week! I didn't always enjoy it at the time but I knew I was learning a huge amount: even three years later I can still remember specific things I learned in those corridors and the patients I examined under pressure. And I know without a doubt that my marks were greatly improved as a result. This, for me, justifies any number of early starts, uncomfortable situations and sweaty shirts. So I would encourage you to pause before dismissing this type of placement – recognise its strengths and potential and challenge yourself to make the most of it while you can.

Placement type A, by contrast, is not a great use of your time, even if it is biscuit Utopia. So you'll be doing your results – and waistline – a favour by recognising this fact and proactively seeking out other learning opportunities, or heading to the library if all else fails. Don't be lulled into thinking a placement is perfect just because it's friendly and comfortable. If you're not learning anything, then the placement is not fulfilling its purpose. Something to consider when filling out your feedback form!

> The major criterion by which to judge a placement should be how much you are learning. Don't be seduced by superficial factors such as the calibre of the facilities or how nice people are: these won't help you pass your exams or become a better doctor!

## 3.4.12 Summary

To summarise everything we've talked about in this section, let's consider what a perfect day might look like on your clinical placements. These have been written for illustrative purposes but draw heavily on my own experiences, and I believe they are realistic and achievable aspirations for students. Not every day will look like this, but hopefully some will!

### The perfect day on a medical placement

08.30: Show up to doctors' office on general medical ward and say hello. Juniors are extremely busy so you quietly grab a copy of the patient list, have a quick skim to see what's happened overnight and quickly look up any relevant results and scans on the computer. You are closely following the case of Mrs Singh in bed 17, so you pop over to say hi and ask how her CT scan went yesterday.

09.00: Ward round begins. The doctors make an effort to involve you, having established that you are enthusiastic and keen to learn. It's a mad rush so you jot down unfamiliar terms like 'MFFD' and 'BIBA' to ask about later.[6] Mr Brown in bed 5 has been admitted with an upper GI bleed from a gastric ulcer – this is totally new to you so you sneak a peek in the Cheese and Onion. The registrar says we'll need to prescribe omeprazole and withhold NSAIDs so you nod sagely and add these to your 'got no idea' list for later. Five interesting new patients have come in overnight so you circle them on your list and resolve to clerk them later. One is a young, healthy-looking bloke who needs a cannula sited – he has big bouncy veins and seems friendly so maybe you could do that this afternoon.

10.30: By the time the round gets to Mrs Singh, the FY1 is so frazzled he can't remember whether she had her CT scan yet or not. You pipe up that yes she had it last night and she has been feeling increasingly nauseous ever since, and hasn't passed urine in 12 hours.

---

6 MFFD = medically fit for discharge. BIBA = brought in by ambulance.

"Ah ha! You're worried about a contrast-induced AKI – great idea!" the consultant says. You nod even more sagely than before, adding a knowing "Mmm… Achey Eye". Discreetly add AKI to your list of topics to look up tonight. The consultant asks for some more blood tests on Mrs Singh. You add these to your potential to-do list for later: she definitely won't shout at you if you mess up taking blood because her son is also studying medicine, so she totally gets it.

11.50: Ward round ends, consultant disappears, junior doctors get busy doing jobs.

11.55: Mainline an espresso.

12.00: Formal teaching on COPD with respiratory consultant. You skimmed this topic over breakfast so the information is familiar to you, even though you don't know it all yet. And you covered inhalers in your self-directed pharmacology learning that week so you muster "dry mouth, tachycardia" when asked about side-effects of salbutamol. Consultant is pleased and doesn't realise you were just describing your own state.

13.00: Lunch. Discuss holiday plans, what's new on Netflix and anything but medicine.

14.00: Back to ward. Consultant nowhere to be seen so juniors finally have time to actually talk to you. FY1 thanks you for helping him out on ward round with Mrs Singh. Registrar talks to you a little more about upper GI bleeds, which seems to be a high-yield topic. She suggests you clerk Mr Brown, look up causes of upper GI bleeding then present the case tomorrow for some informal teaching and to sign off a case-based discussion. You attempt two sets of bloods – one successful, one not, but no worries – and manage the cannula with some help from the FY2. Get a DOP signed off.

15.00: Clerk Mr Brown who turns out to have a systolic murmur, which is cool as you've never heard this before. The other new patients look like they'll be around for a while so there is no rush to clerk them.

15.30: Ward is getting quiet. FY1 tells you to head off, so you go to the library for an hour to look over upper GI bleeds. Decide AKI can wait, but add it to your list to cover later in the week.

16.30: Feeling knackered and already exceeded your limit of five coffees per day so you call it quits. Go for a swim then head out for dinner with friends for a well-deserved evening off.

## The perfect day on a surgery placement

07.00: Eat breakfast while quickly reading up on colorectal cancer and the relevant anatomy for performing an anterior resection procedure. Reflect that you have already come a long way to be able to look at pictures of rectal tumours without ruining your appetite.

07.50: Show up to doctors' office on surgical ward, say hi to the juniors and look at the list to see if anything interesting happened overnight.

08.00: Consultant surgeon shows up for an ultra-fast ward round as she is due in theatres at 08.30. You already asked whether you could join her there, and she seems pleasantly surprised that you actually showed up. See Mr Tan, a 58-year-old who is the first patient on the operating list for today: you already met him in clinic last week after he was referred by his GP under the two-week rule with weight loss and iron deficiency anaemia, which you subsequently read up on. Mr Tan was admitted last night, so you revisited the history and examined him before going home yesterday. He is very anxious about the operation and seems pleased to see you again on ward round.

08.30: Head down to theatres and get changed into scrubs. You and the registrar are the first ones there and nothing much is happening so you ask whether you can briefly present the case to her. She agrees, hears you out, gives you some feedback on your presentation then pulls up Mr Tan's CT scan and blood results and does a bit of informal teaching. She offers to sign off a mini-CEX if you find her later on.

09.00: Consultant arrives and runs through the WHO checklist and introductions. You tell everyone you are a medical student and try to remember all their job titles. Consultant goes to get changed.

09.10: Mr Tan arrives in anaesthetic room. Registrar has disappeared so you say hello to the anaesthetist, who teaches you a little about anaesthetic drugs and lets you insert the cannula.

09.30: Patient unconscious, prepped and ready on the operating table. Surgeon has sensed your enthusiasm and invites you to scrub in. You learned this in clinical skills but it's your first time actually doing it. Fortunately the registrar takes pity on you, reminds you of the different steps and asks a friendly nurse to check you're doing it ok. It takes you eight minutes to scrub in – the consultant and registrar are back at the table in just two. Marvel at how they do that.

09.38: Assist the consultant and registrar with the procedure. You only get to cut sutures and hold various bits of kit but the time absolutely flies by as you are engrossed in the action. They ask you lots of questions about colorectal cancer and definitions of surgical terminology. Both are pleased that you have met Mr Tan and know about his symptoms and scans, and the consultant is dead impressed when you divide your answer about the potential risks of the procedure into immediate, short- and long-term complications.

10.00: Some other medical students show up at the back of the theatre. Surgeon tells them to come back for the next procedure as they have already missed the start of this one. Feel smug.

11.00: The surgeons remove the tumour and you get a clear look at it for the first time. Having felt the lump from the outside, it's fascinating to see what it actually looks like from the inside. You watch them create a stoma and make a mental note to read up on this later. With the procedure almost over, the consultant leaves the registrar to close up and you help by cutting sutures. You thank them both for the teaching and get your mini-CEX signed off.

12.00: Discover you're absolutely starving so head off to get some lunch. Weird how watching surgery does that to you, right? Wonder if deep down you're secretly a cannibal.

13.00: Afternoon procedures didn't sound interesting and you know those other medical students will be jostling for position, so you head to the library for a couple of hours instead. Read up on stomas, update your flashcards and do some practice questions from the surgery section of PassMedicine..

15.00: Head to the ward. There are no other students around and the juniors are pretty free, so you take a set of bloods then clerk and present a patient, leading into a really useful discussion about biliary disease. The patient had hepatomegaly which you admit you hadn't picked up, so the SHO comes back to the bedside and shows you how to improve your technique for palpating and percussing the liver. Mr Tan is now back on the ward: you resolve to see him on the round tomorrow and keep track of his progress.

17.00: Head home. Take a well-deserved evening off from studying and fall asleep in front of **Bake Off**.

# 3.5  The importance of pharmacology

Right, time to stop multi-screening and give me your undivided attention for five minutes. Because I'm going to tell you one of the best things I did at medical school, which was an absolutely crucial factor in my success and can be in yours too.

Pharmacology. Medicines. Drugs and therapeutics. Whatever you call it, you probably shudder a little at the thought of it. You think it's not cool, not fun, not sexy. And perhaps you've got a point. But let me explain why you should devote a massive slice of your time and energy to this topic throughout your clinical years.

Remember how we talked about yield? Well, pharmacology is high yield from the first minute of medical school until the day you retire. It spans all specialties, it's a go-to topic for anyone looking to grill a medical student and it's guaranteed to come up in both written exams and OSCEs. It will make up a huge part of your workload as an FY1, when you're given a lot of responsibility for prescribing and managing drugs. Oh and there's the small matter of the Prescribing Safety Assessment – a national exam you will need to pass before you can qualify (see **Section 5.6**).

**In short, everything you can do to improve your confidence and knowledge of pharmacology is time and effort well spent. By getting on top of it early you'll be doing yourself a huge favour later on, particularly when the PSA rolls around and you can feel smug that you don't need to frantically cram.**

Also, it's very noticeable how easily a strong knowledge of drugs will set you apart from your peers in the early years, whose approach to learning pharmacology will fall somewhere between can't be arsed and really seriously can't be arsed.

So what can you do? Well the first thing is get yourself a copy of one of those clinically focused pharmacology books listed in **Table 3.2** and set about learning it in methodical fashion. You can do this in a group or on your own, as long as you discipline yourself to actually do it. Being geeks, my friends and I set up a study group called Drugs Club (I know, some people were **very** disappointed when they first showed up) to help us do this. Every week we picked five from the **Top 100 Drugs**, for which we would each have to learn the following five facts:

Learn these five facts about any commonly prescribed drug and you'll
be way ahead of the curve:
1.  Indications
2.  Mechanism of action
3.  Side-effects
4.  Warnings
5.  Interactions

This might sound like a lot of work, but it's a nice example of breaking a huge subject down into manageable chunks with clear targets and a structured schedule. Five facts for five drugs equals 25 new facts per week, which is very achievable. And you can make it easier by aligning drugs with other topics you are learning about: for example, on a cardiology week your five drugs could be aspirin, beta blockers, statins, ACE inhibitors and nitrates. At a rate of five per week, you can easily get through a whole pharmacology textbook in an academic year. You almost certainly won't be able to commit everything to memory first time, but don't stress – by even trying, you are already way ahead of the curve.

The second thing you can do to boost your pharmacology knowledge is get into the habit of taking an interest in medications on clinical placements. Any time you hear or see a drug mentioned, write it down in your notebook and resolve to learn the same five key facts about it. Look at drug charts whenever possible, and ask one of the junior doctors if you can talk through all the different drugs with them when they have a few minutes to spare. Even better if you bump into a pharmacist – they *love* talking about drugs and will usually jump at the chance to teach you about them! Patients can also be a great source of information: ask them why they take particular drugs and what side-effects they have experienced. This encourages you to ditch the technical jargon and practise talking about medicines in plain English to lay people. This comes up in OSCEs so the more you can practise, the better. In my finals, for example, we had to explain the mortality benefits of beta blockers to a man with congestive heart failure who was already taking multiple medications and didn't understand why he needed another.

Okay, rant over. I sincerely hope I have persuaded you of the value of pharmacology, even if you now think me even more of a loser than before. Don't delay another minute – start learning those drugs now!

Look through drug charts whenever you get a chance and look up any
medications you are unfamiliar with. Talk about medications with
patients and pharmacists as well as doctors.

# 3.6  Clinical skills, communication skills and OSCEs: level II

In **Chapter 2**, we introduced clinical and communication skills as something you predominantly learn in the classroom and practise on your friends. That was an essential starting point, but now that you're into clinical years it's time to begin putting these skills into practice on real patients in wards and clinics. Placements provide loads of opportunities to do this, particularly as part of bedside teaching and during unstructured ward time.

The main point of examining patients is that they have real signs and symptoms arising from actual pathology. This is your opportunity to find out what crepitations sound like, what splenomegaly feels like and what melaena smells like. Without engaging your senses in this way, these will remain as abstract concepts – just words in a book that are hard to remember. Getting hands-on will also help build up that essential pattern recognition and muscle memory to get faster, slicker and more confident for OSCEs. You won't get there by practising exclusively on your friends, who are usually healthy and therefore boring to examine (it's actually in your best interests to be boring in this context: it was during clinical skills practice that I learned I had tympanosclerosis, then had to endure the next three years of my friends jabbing me with otoscopes to gawp at my eardrums).

**KEY POINT**

There is no substitute for examining and taking histories from real patients. No matter how great your friends are at acting, they can't fake murmurs, ascites or an irregular pulse.

The same principle applies to taking histories. Real people describe things very differently to students or actors who are following a scenario with a particular diagnosis in mind. Real people meander, forget details, get mixed up, use simple words and get fixated on things which might be totally irrelevant to their diagnosis. Only through practice can you learn to navigate this minefield confidently and quickly: to know when to talk and when to listen; when to dwell on a particular point and when to move the conversation forward. You'll also be struck by just how many different diagnoses people have, particularly older patients, which makes their histories much messier than in textbooks.

Your learning curve can start to feel incredibly steep at this point and it is easy to get disheartened, particularly when you 'miss' important signs or pieces of information. This happens to all of us and it's completely natural, so you should expect it to happen and not be downhearted when it does. The solution is to make sure you **learn** from these experiences: if you didn't hear the murmur on a cardiovascular examination, **go back** and listen again, then read up and check out some heart sounds online when you get home. If you thought the cause of someone's blackout was neurological when it was in fact an arrhythmia, **go back** and ask them again how they felt before and after they collapsed, look at the ECG, then make yourself a table later comparing the different presentations of neurological vs. cardiac syncope. Jot down key learning points in your notebook, then look back over them later in the week and ask yourself how you will do things differently next time you examine or take a history from a patient.

> Don't be demoralised when you 'miss' something in a history or examination. Go back to the patient, re-examine or discuss that particular aspect and make sure you learn from it for next time. This will help you build up your pattern recognition.

## 3.6.1 Bedside teaching

Most of the time you'll examine patients on your own or with other students. This is good practice but can make it difficult to get useful feedback on your performance and technique. This is where 'bedside teaching' comes in: these are sessions in which a doctor watches you take a history and examine the patient, then discusses it and gives you feedback afterwards. This can be daunting at first but is, to my mind at least, one of the greatest forms of teaching you'll receive throughout all of medical school.

> Always, always, *always* attend your bedside teaching and sign up to any optional extra or informal sessions you are offered. Write down your feedback and try to take it on board constructively.

Why? Because bedside teaching is the only real forum outside OSCEs in which you get proper, detailed feedback from doctors on your clinical skills. This is invaluable in refining your techniques and drawing attention to things you could do better. And because they're dedicated slots, the teachers have time to spend with you and are fully focused on helping you, especially clinical teaching fellows for whom this is part of their job. If you can't hear the murmur, for example, then now is the time you can admit it without fear of being made to feel stupid. I did that once and the teaching fellow went back to auscultate again, held her stethoscope in the exact spot where the murmur was loudest, handed me the earpieces then stood next to me humming out the murmur ("whoosh-boom, whoosh-boom") until I finally understood what she was on about. I never forgot the sound after that, and instantly became better at recognising it in other patients. This is a level of attention that you will never ever get during a ward round! You can also learn a lot by observing your peers in action and learning from their mistakes too. All of this will help you enormously when faced with the higher-pressure situation of OSCEs.

## 3.6.2 Developing your thinking process

When you first learned how to take a history or perform an examination, it was all about following a rigid series of steps in the correct order, be that presenting complaint through to social history or working anatomically from the arms to the feet. You focused on extracting every last piece of information, without necessarily knowing what to make of it all once you'd extracted it.

This approach has served you nicely as a starting point. But to progress to the next level, you need to start breaking down that rigid structure in order to quickly work out the diagnosis and next steps. When real doctors take histories and examine patients they're not just blindly following a template: every step has a reason behind it and every piece of information they gather serves a specific purpose. Getting to this point will be a long and gradual process, requiring more background knowledge than you probably have yet, but I want you to at least start thinking about it from here on in.

Everyone has their own style but in essence, history taking and examination involves a series of four mental steps (**Box 3.10**). First is a process of elimination. Consider that when you first meet a patient, there are literally **thousands** of potential diagnoses they could have. But each time they answer a question, you can eliminate a whole bunch of those possibilities until only a few remain. I find it helpful to visualise this as a series of funnels through which only a certain number of balls can pass: see **Figure 3.15** for an example using the high-yield scenario of a patient presenting with abdominal pain. Then once you have narrowed it down to a handful of diagnoses, you can proceed to examination: each sign you detect, or don't detect, helps you whittle your list down further until there is only one diagnosis remaining.

Once you have reached a potential diagnosis it's important that you don't just stop there: your diagnosis is only a tentative hypothesis until it's been rigorously tested and other alternatives excluded. So the second

> **How to organise your thinking process during history taking and examination**
>
> 1. Conduct a process of elimination to get you quickly to a hypothesised diagnosis
> 2. Test that hypothesis through focused questioning and examination to strengthen it and thoroughly exclude alternatives
> 3. Once you've settled on a working diagnosis, explore it in more detail
> 4. Go back and fill in the remaining parts of the history and examination you didn't cover yet.

**Box 3.10**

step is to keep gathering more information to strengthen or weaken your hypothesis. This is where you can start to break down that rigid history structure: if you suspect chest pain is cardiac in origin, ask about the major risk factors of smoking and diabetes **straight away** to test your hypothesis, instead of waiting for the past medical and social history sections. If you're suspecting a blood clot, ask promptly about recent travel, surgery and contraceptive use, at the expense of the traditional structure. **Table 3.6** continues the example in our patient with abdominal pain: for this purpose, we'll assume peptic ulcer is our leading diagnosis.

> When hypothesis testing, always bear in mind the most urgent and potentially dangerous differentials. In the case of acute abdominal pain, for example, you need to prioritise excluding appendicitis, GI bleed, ruptured AAA, ovarian torsion and ectopic pregnancy ahead of other diagnoses. These can potentially kill the patient; renal colic, GORD and gallstones almost certainly won't.

**TOP TIP**

Assuming you are now confident with your working diagnosis of peptic ulcer disease, you can move onto stage 3: exploring your diagnosis in more detail. In this stage, you might explore the pattern and nature of the pain further by completing a SOCRATES pain history. This would help you to distinguish between a gastric and duodenal ulcer, the two subtypes of peptic ulcer disease, to make your diagnosis even more specific. You could also use questioning to rule out rarer causes of peptic ulcer disease such as Crohn's disease. Finally, you might ask about any potential complications of peptic ulcer disease, such as bleeding or symptoms of anaemia, as this gives you an idea of severity and how urgently you need to act.[7]

---

7 ALARMS is a helpful mnemonic to run through in suspected peptic ulcer disease to help you pick up any worrying signs which warrant a gastroenterology referral. It stands for Anaemia, Loss of weight, Anorexia, Recent onset or progressive symptoms, Melaena or haematemesis, Swallowing difficulties. Ref: *Oxford Handbook of Clinical Medicine*.

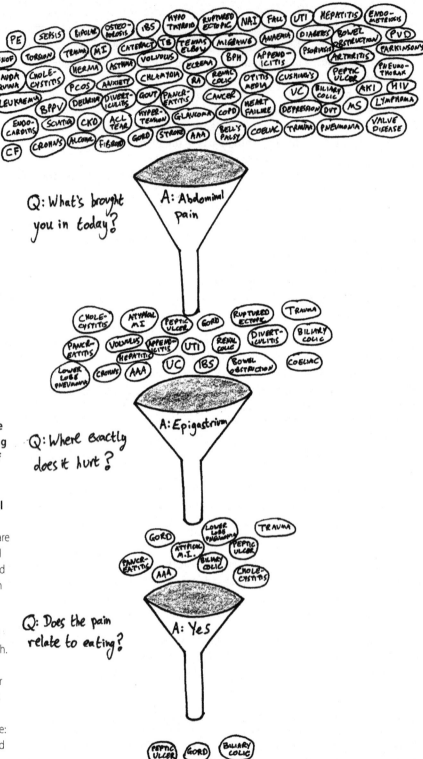

**Figure 3.15: Example of how history taking can act as a series of funnels to narrow down on specific causes of abdominal pain.** When you first meet a patient, there are thousands of potential diagnoses (represented here as balls). But each answer they give to your questions allows only a certain number of balls to pass through. Within just a few questions, the number of potential diagnoses has plummeted from thousands to just three: peptic ulcer, GORD and biliary colic.

**Table 3.6: Example of hypothesis testing in a patient presenting with abdominal pain who you suspect to have peptic ulcer disease.** Keep gathering information to strengthen or weaken your hypothesised diagnosis, even if you have to break down the traditional history structure. If your hypothesis gets stronger you can stick with it. If it gets weaker, you will need to rethink it.

|  | Information that would strengthen your hypothesised diagnosis | Information that would weaken your hypothesised diagnosis |
|---|---|---|
| **History** | Pain worst in epigastrium, burning sensation, comes and goes in association with food or time of day, possibly associated with bloating, belching and reflux<br><br>Relieved by antacids<br><br>History of peptic ulcer disease, previous *H. pylori* infection, NSAID or steroid use and smoking | Pain centred on a different location, constant and unremitting, unrelated to food or time of day, radiates to back, shoulder, groin or iliac fossa, relieved by posture or defecation, associated with dysphagia, weight loss, fevers, dysuria, recurrent vomiting, diarrhoea, constipation, tenesmus, mass or bruising<br><br>History of other GI conditions, autoimmune diseases or alcohol excess |
| **Examination** | Mild epigastric tenderness on palpation, no other specific signs | Cachexia, bruising, palpable mass, Murphy's sign, Rovsing's sign, signs of liver or autoimmune disease, hepato- or splenomegaly |

By now you've reached a diagnosis, hypothesis-tested to exclude alternatives, and explored the diagnosis in more detail. The fourth and final stage is to go back and complete the rest of the history, filling in blanks such as family history, medications or social history. This allows you to build a broader understanding of the patient: their co-morbidities, their lifestyle, the impact the disease is having on them, and so on. This is a very important stage, but note that it comes only once you already have a potential diagnosis in mind, not as the primary information-gathering phase like you were taught in preclinical years. This stage is also useful in an OSCE as you can pick up extra marks for completing these sections of the history.

Developing your thinking pattern in this way takes a lot of time, practice and knowledge. Treat this as a very gradual process and be patient with yourself. If it's making you confused or stressed out during histories and examinations, then just go back to following the original structures until you are more confident to try again later.

**KEY POINT**

### 3.6.3 Improving your history taking

Hopefully the concept of the funnelling process makes sense, even if it seems a lot easier said than done. You're probably thinking it relies on a huge amount of knowledge just to know which questions to ask in the first place, right? Wouldn't it be great if there were some standardised questions you could ask to get the funnelling started with absolutely any presenting complaint?

Well, you're in luck, because there are. Four questions to be precise:[8]

1.  **Have you had this before?**

2.  **Did it come on suddenly or gradually?**

3.  **Is it getting better, worse or staying the same?**

4.  **What were you doing at the time?**

I'm a huge fan of these questions and used them a lot as I progressed through my clinical years. They helped me move on from rigid, ordered history taking to being far more flexible and able to work out the diagnosis much quicker. Ask them at the start of any history: this takes around 30 seconds and instantly gives you a better idea of what's going on with the patient. They're great because they're short and in plain English, so they flow naturally into conversation once the patient has told you their presenting complaint. Used well, they can also give the impression you are listening and responding to the patient, as opposed to the jarring changes of direction that can occur when you follow the classical templates. But behind this friendly veneer, you are extracting some absolutely essential medical information. Here's what the questions are *really* telling you:

1.  **Is this a new problem?**

2.  **Is it acute or chronic?**

3.  **Is it stable or progressive?**

4.  **What are the triggers?**

Pick any presenting complaint, apply these four filters and I guarantee you will substantially whittle down a previously huge list of potential diagnoses. Try it if you don't believe me! The other interesting thing about these questions is just how often you get a positive response to question one. "Oh yes doc, I get this pain all the time. It's my ulcer flaring up. I saw the GP

---

8 Credit to the people at Osler's Room, who taught me the four questions on one of their revision courses.

just last week about it." That's an absolutely massive piece of knowledge which you can easily miss if you don't ask!

History taking is a very personal thing and the four questions approach won't work for everyone. If you like it, then start using it with real patients in plenty of time to get comfortable before OSCEs so you can make it look natural. Ask the four questions at the start, then pause and consider which diagnoses jump to mind in light of the answers, then set about testing your hypotheses by following up on things the patient has said with more specific, focused questions. If you don't like this approach, then come up with your own style: you can use anything provided it is flexible, helps you to get to a diagnosis quickly and develops your thinking patterns in line with **Section 3.6.2**. See **Box 3.11** for some more suggestions.

**How to improve your history-taking skills in the clinical years**

**Box 3.11**

1. Move away from rigid, inflexible structures where you ask a long series of predetermined questions in a predetermined order.
2. Listen carefully to what the patient is telling you, be interested, pick up on their cues and respond to them.
3. Try to reach a working diagnosis quickly, then test it out, then explore it in more detail, then fill in the rest of the history.
4. Have a strong opener such as the four questions to point you in the right direction, after which you can freestyle and be more flexible.
5. Stay calm, friendly and attentive on the outside, no matter how frantically the cogs are whirring on the inside.
6. Always 'ICE' the patient: explore their Ideas, Concerns and Expectations. Do this naturally and empathetically in response to cues; don't just leave it to the end as an afterthought.[9]
7. Vary your pace: use a mix of slow open-ended questions to let the patient talk and quick-fire closed questions to get the information you want.
8. Don't be scared of silence: short pauses can be great for rapport and give both you and the patient some time and space to think.

## 3.6.4 Consolidating your examination skills

Something you can easily start doing from day one of placements is to closely observe real doctors performing examinations on real patients. You will immediately notice that there is a huge variety of style, order and tempo.

---

9 Exploring a patient's ICE means, at a minimum, asking them what *they* think is wrong, whether there is anything they are especially worried about and what they hope to achieve from the consultation. Practise doing this so that you become natural and empathetic, rather than robotically firing through yet more questions.

Often their techniques are very different to what you were taught in your preclinical years and they will instruct you to do it their way. Don't freak out about this! Just smile, nod and do what you're told to avoid conflict. If you like their style, feel free to incorporate it into your own examinations in future, but remember that when it comes to OSCEs it is probably safest to stick to what you were formally taught in medical school because this is usually how mark schemes are constructed. It's also important to stick to what you are confident and comfortable with: if a registrar shows you an awesome technique for accentuating murmurs the week before your OSCE, I would suggest you leave it out until you have practised it enough times to look natural. Better to do the basics really well than try something flashy and make a mess of it!

> **TOP TIP**
>
> Use your first year of clinical placements to get used to examining as many real patients as possible and observing real doctors in action. Don't worry too much about changing your examination techniques just yet: we'll look at how to do this in the next chapter as finals approach.

In the next chapter we'll look at specific ways to tweak your examination skills in preparation for finals: I don't want to overload you just yet as your first clinical year has already given you a vast amount to take in! For now, it's enough to practise your examinations on as many real patients as possible, incorporate any feedback you receive, get used to encountering pathology, build up your pattern recognition and observe real doctors in practice. This approach, coupled with developing your thinking skills and history taking, will put you in a great position for OSCEs in this middle stage of medical school.

> **KEY POINT**
>
> You'll often be asked to perform a 'focused' examination on clinical placements. This is medical code for 'quick, realistic and sensible', as opposed to the lengthy, sprawling examinations you were taught in preclinical years. If someone has pneumonia, for example, focus on auscultating their chest instead of looking for clubbing and Horner's syndrome. If they've presented with abdominal pain, go straight to their abdomen rather than looking for angular stomatitis or leukonychia. This lets you focus on pathology, pattern recognition and diagnostic skills. It makes examination a lot quicker and more enjoyable in the process!

## 3.6.5 Evolving your practice sessions

As well as getting used to real patients, it's essential to keep practising your clinical and communication skills with your friends and running mock OSCEs, particularly as end-of-year exams approach. This maintains your muscle memory and allows you to practise skills which you didn't get an opportunity to use on placements. But try to gradually evolve these sessions to be more reflective of real-life practice and the sort of stations that might come up in OSCEs between now and finals (see **Section 4.5.7** for specifics). Here are some of the ways you can do this:

- **Use a wide range of OSCE resources:** see *Table 3.2*. Anything labelled 'for finals' is appropriate from here on in, even if finals are still a couple of years away.

- **Include pathology:** the 'patient' can try to fake certain symptoms and signs, draw scars or bruises on themself, tell you out loud what you're supposed to be finding, show you pictures or videos or play you audio of heart or lung sounds. Be creative! It's not as good as the real thing but it's a darned sight better than nothing.

- **Focus on getting the diagnosis:** now that you're in the groove of basic histories and examinations, you can work on refining your thinking process and history-taking skills, as discussed in **Sections 3.6.3** and **3.6.4**. Start to move away from rote rehearsal to a more flexible and realistic style which lets you figure out what's going on.

- **Present your findings and top three differentials to an imaginary examiner:** get in the habit of *always* doing this after an examination. Limit yourself to one minute and constructively critique each other's presentations.

- **State which further examinations are required:** this step is easily missed and can cost you marks in an OSCE. Practise saying "To complete my examination, I would like to examine the joint above and below", or the cardiovascular system, or the hernial orifices, or whatever else is relevant.

- **Show your working:** personally I see no harm in a small amount of 'thinking out loud', such as stating *why* you think certain differentials are more or less likely than each other. This helps you organise your thoughts and shows the examiner your thinking process, which can boost their overall impression even if you got the answer wrong.

- **Suggest next steps:** elaborate on your list of differentials by suggesting which investigations you would like to do next to rule the diagnosis in or out. Don't just randomly throw things out there: you should know exactly why you are doing each test and how you would act on the results (see **Box 3.12**).

- **Have a reasonable idea about management:** you're not really expected to know the detailed management of every condition just yet, but it certainly helps to know at least some of the basics. Practise stating out loud how you'd like to manage the patient once the diagnosis is confirmed.

- **Introduce exam-style questions:** after listening to the summary, the examiner should ask the student a few 'viva-style' questions to explore their knowledge. This is a good habit to get into, whether or not your medical school includes these in OSCEs. Most role-play scenarios come with a few questions provided, or you can write your own.

**Box 3.12**

**E-BOXES**

This is a brilliant mnemonic for presenting the investigations you would like to do next when summing up at the end of an OSCE station. It's systematic and ensures you don't forget anything.

    **E** = Examination (if you haven't done it already)[10]

    **B** = Blood tests

    **O** = Orifices: swabs, urine, sputum and stool tests

    **X** = X-rays and other imaging

    **E** = ECG

    **S** = Special tests: everything else

---

10 The first E is absolutely vital: it's surprisingly easy in a history station to forget that you've not examined the patient and go straight onto discussing blood tests, which makes you look silly. I did this in finals and failed the station mostly as a result: it was one of only two stations I failed in all of medical school! And it was precisely because I didn't do E-BOXES!

## 3.6.6 The Big Three investigations: CXRs, ECGs and ABGs

In **Sections 3.2** and **3.3** we talked about how you should be shifting the content of your studies away from abstract scientific concepts and onto more clinically focused topics. Among the most important of these is interpreting investigations, which you should devote a lot of time and attention to. Hopefully you'll get plenty of practice on placements and during SDL, but it is also worth incorporating investigations into your clinical skills practice because they start to come up a lot in OSCEs (**Figure 3.16**).

Common blood tests such as FBC, U&Es, LFTs, TFTs, bone profile, coagulation and CRP are all essential to understand, as well as urine dip results, spirometry and abdominal X-rays. However, there is a 'Big Three' which we will focus on, because they're the ones you will most commonly be asked to present and interpret: chest X-rays, ECGs and arterial blood gases.

As with most things in medicine, it helps enormously in these situations to have a structured framework you can work through. These investigations contain potentially huge amounts of information, and you need to be systematic to ensure you don't miss anything. There are lots of different frameworks in circulation, but some examples are given in **Boxes 3.13–3.15**.

Practise going through these with your friends, taking it in turns to stand up and work through a whole example under timed conditions. Do this as often as possible until it starts to flow naturally and you can remember the different sections effortlessly. This will be invaluable in

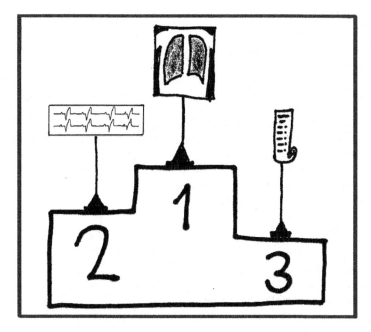

Figure 3.16: Chest X-rays, ECGs and arterial blood gases come up a lot in written exams and OSCEs. Make sure you are comfortable interpreting and presenting them out loud.

OSCEs, as they often spring these investigations on you right at the end of a station when you are already mentally frazzled and running out of time. It helps enormously if you can whizz through your framework quickly, efficiently and systematically, using the minimum amount of brainpower.

**TOP TIP**

When presenting an ECG or CXR, state the most obvious abnormality first, before going through your systematic approach in more detail. Otherwise you can look silly by talking about airways and bones before mentioning that whopping great lung cancer staring you in the face.

**Box 3.13**

**A structured framework for presenting and interpreting chest X-rays:**

1. **Basics:** note the patient's name, when the X-ray was taken, whether it's erect or supine and PA or AP
2. **State any glaringly obvious findings**
3. **Comment on image quality:** RIPE
    Rotation: are the clavicles aligned?
    Inspiration: how many ribs can you see?
    Penetration: are the spinous processes clearly visible?
    Exposure: does it look particularly dark or bright?
4. **ABCDE approach:**
    Airway
    Bones, Breasts and soft tissues
    Cardiac outline, Cardiophrenic and Costophrenic angles
    Diaphragm
    Effusions
    lung Fields
    Great vessels
    Hila
    overall Impression

**Box 3.14**

**A structured framework for presenting and interpreting ECGs:**

1. **Basics:** note the patient's name, when the ECG was taken and whether it's correctly calibrated and set to the correct speed
2. **State any glaringly obvious findings**
3. **Comment systematically on:**

    | | |
    |---|---|
    | 1. Axis | 6. PR interval |
    | 2. Rhythm | 7. QRS complexes |
    | 3. Heart rate | 8. ST segments |
    | 4. P waves | 9. T waves |
    | 5. Is it sinus rhythm? | 10. QT interval |

4. **Give your overall impression**

**A structured framework for presenting and interpreting blood gases:**

Box 3.15

1. **Basics:** note the patient's name, date and time the sample was taken, whether it's arterial or venous and how much oxygen the patient was on at the time
2. **Check pH:** state whether there is acidosis (pH <7.35), alkalosis (pH >7.45) or normal pH
3. **Check oxygenation:** is the patient hypoxic ($PO_2$ <8kPa)? If so, state whether it is type 1 ($PCO_2$ <6kPa) or type 2 ($PCO_2$ >6kPa) respiratory failure
4. **Check $PCO_2$:** does it explain the pH? Carbon dioxide is acidic so if it's high (>6), that would explain an acidosis; if it's low (<4.7), that would explain an alkalosis. Both patterns are consistent with a primary respiratory problem. If $PCO_2$ is inconsistent with the pH then it is a compensatory change.
5. **Check $HCO_3^-$:** does it explain the pH? Bicarbonate is alkaline so if it's high (>26), that would explain an alkalosis; if it's low (<22) that would explain an acidosis. Both patterns are consistent with a primary metabolic problem. If $HCO_3^-$ is inconsistent with the pH then it is a compensatory change.
6. **One-line summary:** state whether it is a: respiratory/metabolic/mixed ... acidosis/alkalosis ...with full/partial/no compensation
7. **Suggest possible causes:** if there is a metabolic acidosis, check the anion gap. If this is increased you can use the mnemonic KULT, which covers all the main possibilities.[11] If it's not a metabolic acidosis then ignore the anion gap and work logically through conditions that could increase or decrease carbon dioxide or bicarbonate (whichever is the primary cause).

## 3.6.7 Having station titles in advance

One of the ways medical schools have tried to get around the issue of students cheating is to release station 'titles' a couple of days in advance of OSCEs. These tend to be brief and fairly generic, such as "musculoskeletal examination" or "procedural skills". Sometimes they give a little more information about the tasks expected of you, such as: "neurological history, interpreting results with diagnosis and management plan". Occasionally they are deliberately vague: in finals, we had "common primary care examination", which could have been pretty much anything but turned out to be a breast examination.

---

11 KULT: Ketones, Urea, Lactate, Toxins (salicylates, methanol, ethylene glycol)

The aim of this approach is to level the playing field: by giving everyone this information, the cheaters' advantage is supposedly taken away. And the med school can continue to mix up the patients, pathology and diagnoses to ensure you still have to think on your feet and prove yourself, even if you know roughly what's coming. I thought about this a lot but never really reached an opinion about whether it's a good idea or not. You could persuade me either way! Anyway it really doesn't matter: if your medical school does this then you will have to live with it, regardless of your or my view on it as an anti-cheating strategy.

**TOP TIP**

If your med school releases station titles before your OSCEs, be sure to get together with some friends and brainstorm every possibility to ensure you are ready for anything. This is an extremely worthwhile exercise which should take priority over everything else on your revision timetable!

If you are faced with this approach then I would strongly encourage you to get together with a group of friends as soon as the station titles are released. Brainstorm every possibility that could come up, make sure you have practised them all and feel confident to at least make a good go of them. In particular, rehearse the examinations over and over so that your muscle memory and fluency come back, which will free up brain space on the day to consider differentials and next steps. It's important to do this process in a group because people will come up with ideas you didn't think of, prompting you to cover bases you would otherwise have missed. For example, I had somehow convinced myself that "common primary care examination" was going to be otoscopy or fundoscopy, and it was only thanks to my friends that I was nudged to revise breast examination!

Of course you still need to keep an open mind on the day and be adaptable – don't let your heart sink when the station turns out not to be what you thought – but in my opinion you'd be mad not to at least consider all the options in advance. It's completely fair game and everyone else will be doing it, so don't disadvantage yourself!

## 3.6.8  Summary

In this section, we have looked at tips to help you through the second phase of developing your clinical and communication skills for placements and OSCEs. The key points are:

- Real patients are amazing – start examining and taking histories from them as much as you can, not just from your friends.
- Attend bedside teaching. It's the bomb. You'll get great feedback.
- Start to develop your thinking process so you can quickly get to a hypothesised diagnosis, test it, explore it in more detail then fill in the rest of the history.
- Don't be demoralised when this turns out to be much easier said than done!
- Work on your history-taking skills: move away from long predetermined lists of questions to a more flexible approach.
- Observe how real doctors examine patients.
- Build up your recognition of clinical signs.
- Evolve your OSCE practice sessions to reflect the more complex stations they will start to throw at you.
- Practise using E-BOXES and structured frameworks for presenting chest X-rays, ECGs and ABGs.
- If OSCE station titles are released in advance, put in a serious shift of brainstorming with your mates to figure out and prepare for all the possibilities.

# 3.7　Thinking ahead: bits and bobs

At the end of a long and exhausting first year of clinical placements, it's probably too early for most students to be seriously considering the Foundation Programme or future careers, so we will leave those to later chapters. However, there are a few useful things to think about at this stage of medical school:

- Consider carefully whether to intercalate, if you have this option. Pros: more points for Foundation Programme applications, chance to beef up your CV for future careers, have a potentially relaxed year to break up the madness of clinical placements. Cons: adds another year to your degree, builds up more debt, drops you behind your original year group.

- Get involved with any publications, audits or quality improvement projects that come your way. Publications get you extra points for Foundation Programme applications; audits and QIPs may help you with specialty training applications.

- Decide what you want to get out of any SSCs/SSMs (student-selected components/modules) this year or next. If your goal is to enhance your CV, then choose something that fits your intended specialty and looks and sounds impressive, such as shadowing a neurosurgeon at Queen Square. If your goal is to relax, choose something less taxing like mindfulness or building sculptures out of medical supplies.

- Try to keep up your passion and interest for medicine, instead of letting all that exam and OSCE stress drain it out of you. Go to talks and exhibitions, watch documentaries and TV shows like **Hospital**, listen to podcasts like **Sharp Scratch** and **Inside Health**, read books like **This is Going to Hurt**, **Do No Harm**, and **The House of God** and absolutely anything by Atul Gawande. Everything you can do to enjoy medicine in its fullest will help keep you enthusiastic and fresh for the years ahead.

- If you **are** lucky enough to already have firm ideas about what you want to do, then sneak a peek ahead to **Section 4.6** for some more pointers. In particular, check out the 'person specifications' for your chosen specialty: some are extremely competitive and you may be able to get ahead by having merits, distinctions and prizes. This may require you to rethink your work ethic for this year and next!

- Listen out for any upcoming changes to medical education which may affect you in later years. At the time of writing, for example, the GMC had announced plans to introduce a new UK Medical Licensing Assessment (UKMLA) which all graduates will have to pass from 2022 to practise in the UK.[12,13] Details are currently too thin on the ground for me to go into this, but depending on when you are reading this book you may need to figure it out and prepare accordingly!

12 *BMJ* 2017;358:j2227
13 www.gmc-uk.org/education/standards-guidance-and-curricula/projects/medical-licensing-assessment

# Chapter 4
# Second clinical year

## Contents

# 4.1 What's it all about?

Congratulations on surviving your first clinical year. It's a huge achievement. You've started getting used to the hospital environment, to interacting with real patients and to learning on the job alongside actual doctors. You've also discovered that there is an alarm clock function on your phone, that shirts need to be ironed and that hangovers and ward rounds are a **terrible** combination. Your transformation into a junior doctor is now well under way.

That's the good news. The bad news is that the really difficult part starts now. Because, in my experience at least, the second clinical year was the hardest and longest of all of medical school. Mainly because of the sheer volume of information you're expected to cover: as we will see shortly, you're going to have **entire specialties** thrown at you in rapid succession with no breathing space in between. It's also a very important year because finals are now firmly on the horizon, and people will start to expect more from you as you approach the finish line. And remember: it's your last chance to boost your academic marks before submitting your Foundation Programme application, as final year usually doesn't count.

This is not meant to scare you: although tough, I also found it a very satisfying year, full of amazing learning opportunities and experiences which shaped my ideas about medicine and prepared me for becoming a doctor. Being exposed to such a broad range of different specialties in quick succession kept things interesting and exciting, as my placements were never long enough to get boring. This exposure also allows you to start imagining yourself as a doctor for perhaps the first time, and to develop ideas about where you want your career to go. It might even inspire you to pick a specialty and start developing your CV towards it. So despite being long and difficult it was an extremely worthwhile and satisfying year in the end. I look back fondly on it – I hope that you will too!

**TOP TIP**

> Your second clinical year can be long and exhausting, particularly if you are rotating through new specialties every few weeks. Pace yourself, look after yourself and make extra sure you are studying efficiently, effectively and using your time wisely.

Before getting into the nitty gritty, we must clarify some details so you can work out exactly what does and doesn't apply to your medical school. For me, this was my third year of a four-year degree and it was called P-year, short for penultimate year. It was composed almost entirely of clinical placements: the only university time was the odd week of introductory lectures and workshops before beginning each placement.

The really big difference between P-year and the previous clinical year was the introduction of 'specialty' placements: psychiatry, neurology, paediatrics and obstetrics and gynaecology. Lasting five weeks each, these were the only clinical placements we had for these specialties throughout all of medical school, making it a very tall order to cover all the material (some universities provide more exposure than this – it's common to have two separate placements for psych, paeds and O&G, for example). There were also general medical and general surgical placements, just like the year before, but with more sub-specialisation this time around, including placements in ENT, orthopaedics, urology, breast surgery, ophthalmology, plastics, cardiology, geriatrics, acute medicine and palliative care.

So in this chapter we will focus on these **specialties,** as distinct from general medicine and general surgery placements: in particular, how you can get to grips with an entire specialty in just five weeks, and how to incorporate specialties into your clinical skills and OSCE practice. We'll also look at developing your SDL in preparation for finals, how to enhance your examination and presentation skills and how to take your pharmacology knowledge to the next level. For the purposes of this chapter, we'll leave the university setting behind us and assume you're now based entirely on clinical placements.

# 4.2 Techniques

Penultimate year can be a tricky time for your studies and many students feel their momentum start to falter. You've already tried and tested all your techniques and are probably getting a little bored of some of them. Yet there's a stronger need than ever for self-motivation to study, as almost all your learning takes place on clinical placements now, with precious little classroom and lecture time in between. You won't necessarily have a structured timetable telling you exactly which topics to cover at what time. This doesn't suit everyone: it can be especially challenging if you are just returning from an intercalated degree year, where your tasks were very clearly defined for you and the shorter hours allowed life to go back to relaxation mode. And to compound matters, your friends may now be scattered around different hospitals or even in different years, which breaks up your revision groups and takes away some of the impetus to study. These feelings are entirely natural and you can turn them into a positive thing by recognising and addressing them, rather than just muddling through and hoping for the best.

**It's important not to falter or burn out at this stage, when you've already come so far and the finish line is almost in sight.**

The key, I think, is to set your expectations properly and be honest and realistic with yourself about what does and doesn't work for you. Bring together all of the study skills you have learned so far and push yourself to do things better, smarter and more efficiently, not just harder, longer or in larger quantities. If writing notes has become a chore, for example, then don't waste time on them: move on to another technique which helps the information stick better in less time. If you find yourself constantly exhausted and having nightmares about ECGs: take a proper break, re-think your time management strategies and carve out more me-time to balance out the studying. If you hate sitting in clinics, then don't punish yourself with them: stick to other activities you enjoy and actually learn from. It's a long year with a vast amount of information to process: you will need to keep yourself fresh and engaged if you are to make it through to finals with your sanity intact!

## 4.2.1 How to blitz an entire specialty in five weeks

If your medical degree is anything like mine, then the unrelenting pace of specialties year will present an absolutely fearsome challenge. You were given months or even years to learn general medicine and surgery – now they're flinging entire specialties at you every five or six weeks. I'm not exaggerating: I've gone back and checked my timetable and we were given a measly five-week placement to cover **the whole of obstetrics and gynaecology** (plus a piddling three days of intro lectures). It's bonkers – a woman gets 40 weeks to grow a foetus, yet in **one-eighth** of that time we're supposed to learn absolutely everything about her pregnancy from conception right through to delivery and the postnatal period? And that's just the O half of O&G – there's an entire complex world of vaginas, menstrual cycles and contraception to top that all off. And don't even get me started on paediatrics: five weeks to learn **everything that can go wrong with a child between birth and age 18**? I mean seriously, what were they smoking when they devised these timetables?

Backed into a corner like this, you have no choice but to come out fighting. Your med school has basically thrown down a gauntlet: are you up to the challenge of learning an entire specialty to finals standard in just five weeks? The answer is a resounding **hell yes you are**. To prove it, you will need to wage war on these specialties and loot the spoils of knowledge. Here's how.[1]

## Phase I: reconnaissance (two weeks)

Start by splitting the placement into separate phases of two and three weeks. The first phase is all about information gathering and strategising. Essentially, you need to put time and effort into identifying and prioritising the high-value topics that are most likely to come up in your exams, because you simply cannot afford to waste time on anything else. To do this, you will need to take a bird's-eye view of the entire landscape and focus on identifying the high-yield topics you want to target (**Figure 4.1**). To keep track, I'd suggest making a list of topics, either on paper or in a Word document, so that you can continually rank and prioritise them in order as you go along. Be ruthless with low-yield topics that don't make the cut.

That's the principle, now here's how to go about it:

1.  **Look carefully over the intro lectures.** You're being scattered to different hospitals for placements, so the med school can't be sure you will all have the same experience. The communal intro lectures are therefore the most consistent teaching on which it is fairest to test everyone. Although a less reliable resource than in preclinical years, it remains more likely than not that exam questions will be drawn from these slides.

2.  **Attend clinical tutorials and bedside teaching.** Your medical school will help you out by ensuring your in-placement teaching focuses on the most important, need-to-know topics (they're presumably trying to make amends for shafting you with the timetable). Between these and the lecture slides, you should be able to figure out what you need to focus on.

3.  **Immerse yourself in the placement.** Show up loads, jot down which patients and conditions you encounter and note how doctors talk about them. Lots of patients = high-yield condition (unless you

---

1 I developed this approach for coping with neurology, psychiatry, paediatrics and O&G, but you could apply it to any placement in any specialty.

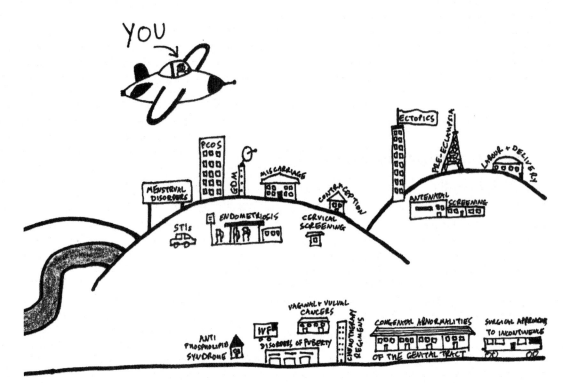

**Figure 4.1: The two-week reconnaissance phase involves taking a bird's-eye view of the entire specialty so you can decide how to prioritise your studies.** Think of yourself as having arrived in an unfamiliar land, and you are scouting out the territory to identify the most important targets to neutralise. In this example, using O&G, the high-yield topics are shown on the highlands and low-yield on the lowlands.

are on a super-specialty unit); isolated case = low yield. Listen out for phrases like 'classic case' or 'common presentation' – go clerk that patient and commit them to memory!

4. **Smash through online question banks and MCQ books.** This is the time to prioritise quantity over quality: try to get through as many practice questions as you can, purely to get a feel for which topics come up most regularly and carry the most marks. Update your topics list accordingly.

5. **Do not worry about getting these questions wrong for now.** I know we are perfectionists but seriously, do not give even *one ounce* of a crap because at this stage you are just scouting and gathering information, not testing yourself. In fact getting them wrong is useful as it helps establish how good your baseline knowledge is. You can reset your scores later, so just ignore your homepage telling you you're a bottom-decile loser.

6.  **Ask the specialty trainees.** They'll almost certainly be able to tell you which are the most important topics you need to know about for finals. Juniors are usually better to ask than consultants, for whom med school finals are a very distant memory. Consultants may also have a skewed view towards rare and unusual things which they find interesting. You need to prioritise common, everyday stuff.

7.  **Look at the LOBs.** But don't stress about them. I barely used them at this stage. It's better to figure out the key topics for yourself.

8.  **Calibrate knowledge.** Gauge what your fellow students know and consider important, especially those who have already done the placement.

9.  **Skim textbooks.** Don't go deep into topics yet – just try to get a feel for which ones seem to be given the most priority. See **Table 4.4** for some suggested reading.

10. **Look up the latest guidelines.** Bear in mind that stuff you learned earlier in medical school may already be out of date, so you don't want to waste time going over it again. For the purposes of exams, whatever's in the latest guideline is always correct (unless the medical school hasn't got around to updating the questions, which would be a serious oversight and you'd be within your rights to complain).

11. **Be aware of any controversy or conflicts.** These are useful to know about for placements and for showing off in OSCEs, but are essentially off limits for MCQs (hooray!). If the world's leading experts can't agree on the management of a particular condition, they can hardly expect medical students to be definitive about it!

## Reconnaissance phase: example

It's vital for the learning process that you identify the high-yield topics for yourself, so I'm not going to just tell you what they are (I know, I'm such a meanie). However, let's stick with O&G and look at one example from early in my placement which I remember very well: I spent a morning in clinic with a super-nice and enthusiastic urogynaecologist who talked at length about surgical approaches to prolapse and stress urinary incontinence, including the pros and cons of colposuspension, slings and surgical tape/ mesh. I knew nothing about urogynaecology at the time and found it really interesting (the use of surgical tape/mesh turns out to be very topical and controversial, and has received a lot of media coverage). I left with the impression that I needed to know about the surgical management of urogynaecological prolapse and urinary incontinence in quite some detail.

Rather than rushing to read up or make notes on it, I added it to my list of potential subjects for later. When I spent some time looking back over the intro lectures and whizzing through practice questions, I established that urinary incontinence and prolapse are indeed high-yield topics, being common and potentially very distressing conditions. However, the details of specific surgical approaches were low yield and unlikely to come up in my exams – I decided it was enough just to know that there **are** surgical approaches, the very basics of what they entail and when they can be considered. Ultimately, I reduced all of urogynaecology to just six high-yield, need-to-know essentials. Here they are, as they appeared in my end-of-placement electronic flashcards:

1. Define stress urinary incontinence. What are the most common causes?

2. What is the management of stress urinary incontinence? (brief overview of conservative, medical and surgical approaches).

3. Define urge urinary incontinence. What are the most common causes? In particular, what is overactive bladder syndrome and how is it diagnosed?

4. What is the management of overactive bladder syndrome? (brief overview of conservative, medical and surgical approaches).

5. What are the different types and degrees of pelvic organ prolapse, and what causes it?

6. What is the management of pelvic organ prolapse? (brief overview of conservative, medical and surgical approaches).

If you can answer these six flashcards, then you've got urogynaecology covered for finals, including OSCEs. It's entirely possible you could face an OSCE station where you take a history from a woman who is suffering from incontinence, and you are expected to establish whether it is stress or urge and counsel her on treatment options accordingly (top tip: a kindly manner and exploration of the impact on her life would be essential in an incontinence history). You will not have a station where a woman has already failed conservative and medical approaches to stress incontinence and you need to talk her through the relative merits of a sling procedure compared to a mesh insertion. That's a surgeon's job!

Use the reconnaissance phase to work out how much you need to know, and give yourself the confidence to prioritise accordingly. Don't dive into studying a topic just because it happened to come up that day, or because a consultant told you to – if you decide it's low yield then show it no mercy when planning your studies.

## Phase II: all-out assault (three weeks)

Now you've figured out what the key topics are in your specialty, you need to get head down, bum up and start learning the stuff. You've only got three weeks left to do this so you will need to strike hard and fast, deploying all of the study techniques and time management skills you have learned so far into multiple lines of attack (**Figure 4.2**, **Box 4.1**). Don't leave it until revision time – when you've got to learn an entire specialty in such a short space of time, there really is no alternative but to learn the material as you go along. You should devote some proper time to this and aim to learn **as much as you can** during the placement itself, as this will make life vastly easier when it comes to revision period.

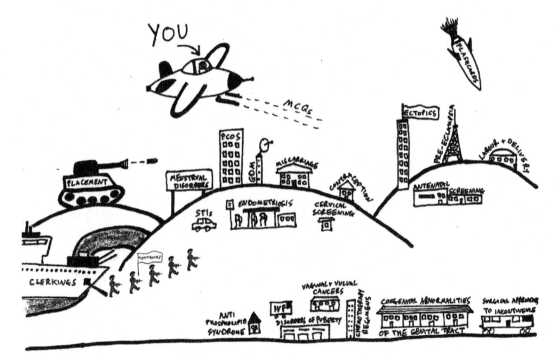

Figure 4.2: Once you have identified the high-yield topics, spend the next three weeks laying waste to them using all of the different study techniques and resources we have discussed so far. Challenge yourself to learn as much as you can about these topics in the time you have left, being extra efficient with your time. Leave the low-yield topics unscathed!

Be extra efficient with your time on placement during phase II: only show up to clinics and ward rounds if you're learning things; make your excuses and leave if you aren't. If you find juniors who are keen to teach informally then make friends with them, buy them coffee and try to get maximum educational value from them. If the placement has run dry then head to the library and be disciplined with your time there. On the plus side, now that you're into the second half of the placement it should be easier to skive off as you've already made a good impression by showing your face plenty in the first couple of weeks.

**Box 4.1**

### Top tips for phase II: all-out assault

Use these in addition to all the other techniques and resources we have discussed throughout this book.

- Match your study topics to placement activities. For example, if you've put allergy on your list of key paediatrics topics: do some pre-reading, go along to allergy clinic, ask questions, examine kids and talk to their parents. Spend a couple of hours consolidating and reinforcing that knowledge afterwards and hey presto – that's paediatric allergy done in a day. Cross it off your list.

- Try to learn at least five things from every patient you clerk. You can't afford to waste time on clerkings you don't learn from. If the patient has a high-yield condition, turn them into a self-contained learning case by reviewing every aspect from presentation through to investigations and management, and making good notes or flashcards afterwards.

- Use case study/clinical scenario books in your SDL time for specialties like paediatrics, psychiatry, neurology and O&G (*Section 4.3.1*). Working through a whole case from the beginning really hones your thinking process and is great for OSCEs, particularly if you have long cases. MCQs alone won't do this.

- Electronic flashcards *really* come into their own now, as spaced repetition is a perfect method for learning things in a short time frame. Give it a go if you've not tried it yet. Build a deck for each placement, so you've got it ready to dip straight back into when exams are approaching.

- If you have to write up cases or present at student grand round, always pick a patient with a high-yield disease. This is efficient use of time, as preparing your presentation doubles up as SDL.

- As you progress through phase II, reset your scores on your online MCQ bank then start doing the questions again, going through the explanations in more detail. Hopefully you'll get more questions right now, as you've actually covered the material beforehand.

## Phase III: survey the aftermath (half a day)

At the very end of each block, take a good look back over your topics list and spend a few hours making a set of notes to yourself, keeping track of which topics you covered properly and which you didn't get around to (**Figure 4.3**). Note which resources you found useful, any memorable patients you encountered or experiences you had, and take stock of where your strengths and weaknesses lie. Save this document somewhere you can easily find it again.

This will be an absolutely **huge** help when exam revision comes around because, realistically, you will be too busy on other placements to look at these topics much before then (although of course you should try to do so!). If your paediatrics placement was in September, say, it will feel like a distant memory by exam time in May–June, and you'll be extremely grateful to yourself for having this kind of information handy so you can try to pick up where you left off.

> At the end of a specialty placement, organise your ideas and resources so that you can pick things up where you left off when revision period rolls around. All that hard work is wasted if the information just fades from your brain and you have to start again from scratch.

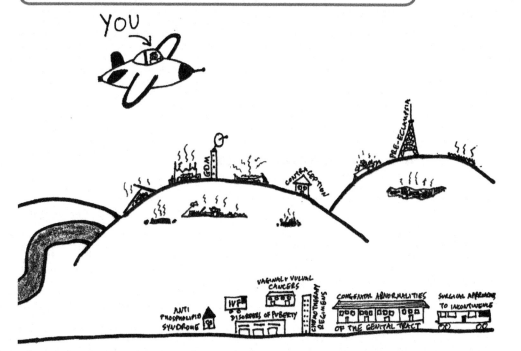

**Figure 4.3: Surveying the aftermath of your learning is an absolutely essential step once your specialty placement draws to an end.** Take note of which topics you tackled properly (shown here as smouldering rubble) and which you didn't get around to (left unscathed). Write down pointers for your future self. This will be absolutely invaluable when revision period comes around, as it saves you having to start again from scratch.

## 4.2.2 **Grab extra learning opportunities**

Have you ever sat opposite a convicted murderer and listened to them gleefully brag about how they killed their victim, without showing the merest hint of compassion or regret? I have. It's a disturbing, deeply unsettling experience, which will stay with me forever.

This was just one of many memorable and uncomfortable moments on a visit to Broadmoor Hospital, the UK's most famous high-security psychiatric hospital. We went as part of our psychiatry placements, to give us a taster of forensic psychiatry. I also visited a prison, a psychiatric intensive care unit and an inpatient eating disorders unit, each of which challenged me in different ways. That was on psychiatry; in neurology I spent a day at a rehabilitation hospital meeting patients recovering from major strokes, in O&G I sat in on termination clinics and in palliative care I visited a hospice to talk to dying patients and their families.

Each of these trips, and the patients I met, lodged deep in my memory, giving me insights to these subspecialties that no lecture or textbook ever could. On a personal level, I also found these visits moving, challenging and – yes, it sounds clichéd – inspirational. If your med school offers similar opportunities, I would implore you to grab them because you may never get these chances again. They can shape your ideas about medicine, humanity, your career and the world around you. Get on top of your studies to ensure you can spare the time, then sign up to as much stuff as you can. You'll feel very far out of your comfort zone at times but you'll learn an enormous amount and, to my mind at least, be a better and more compassionate doctor as a result.

## 4.2.3 **Work towards finals**

Something important to keep in mind during your second clinical year is that you are now essentially working towards a finals-level of knowledge, despite not actually being in your final year yet. Because, as we will see in the next chapter, final year isn't really about expanding your knowledge: it's predominantly about consolidating the stuff you already know and getting you ready for the Foundation Programme. So it's helpful to view penultimate year as the time to build up to the peak of your knowledge, and final year as simply a bonus on top. *Box 4.2* tells you what this means in practical terms.

**What are the practical implications of being one year away from finals?**

- You need to work hard this year. Sorry!
- You will have to learn **a *lot*** of new information.
- Almost the entire curriculum will be examinable this year, so don't put subjects off for next year.
- Start using resources and questions that are labelled 'for finals': this is the level you are aiming at now.
- If you're doing a placement for the last time, be aware you're not going to get any more teaching or placements on it in final year but will still be examined on it, so now's the time to get your head around the material properly.
- If there are any resources or techniques you didn't try yet, now's the time!
- You can help out your future self by creating top-quality learning resources to come back to when finals revision time comes around.
- You can still make some subtle but important adjustments to the ways you study: we'll look at these in *Sections 4.2.4–4.2.6*.

## 4.2.4 Integrate your academic study with clinical and communication skills

One of the most important concepts to understand if you're to survive this year and prepare yourself for finals is how to integrate your studies in a way that prepares you for written exams and OSCEs *at the same time*.

In the early years of medical school, you were almost certainly taught in a very compartmentalised way. You had academic subjects like anatomy, physiology and pathology, then your clinical and communication skills programme ran alongside. These subjects might have aligned in time, for example learning lower limb anatomy in the same week as learning how to perform a knee examination, but I bet they were otherwise separate. At no point did the anatomy teacher, pathologist and clinical skills tutor get together to put on a combined session covering everything you need to know about the knee.

As a result, these subjects end up somewhat separate in your brain and during your study sessions: when practising clinical skills with your

Early in medical school, you are taught in 'silos' such as anatomy, clinical examination, radiology and so on. As you move towards finals you will need to break down these artificial barriers and bring this knowledge all together.

**KEY POINT**

**TOP TIP** Start integrating your academic studies with your clinical and communication skills. Any time you are studying one aspect of a disease, make an effort to consider all the others.

friends, for example, you might have examined the knee, the shoulder and the lumbar spine in a single session, before chucking in a random cardiovascular or abdo exam if you had time. It's less likely you would have stuck with the knee for a whole session in which you practised knee examination and history taking from people with knee pain, then revised knee anatomy, then brainstormed all the different pathologies affecting the knee, reviewed knee X-rays and joint aspiration cytology, before finally discussing treatment options for knee problems.

Until now that has been absolutely fine. That's how medicine is taught, and in the early years it makes sense. But if you really think about it, it's actually a bit weird and unrepresentative of how real medicine is practised. Say you're a person with knee pain – you will go to your GP or an A&E doctor and expect them to do **all of the above**, referring to other specialties only when necessary. You don't expect the GP to send you to an anatomist for the examination, then to an exercise physiologist for dynamic testing, a radiologist for imaging and a rheumatologist for joint aspiration, before eventually sending you to the orthopaedic surgeon to have your ACL tear repaired.

So at some point in your training you need to evolve from the medical student who holds everything in separate mental silos into the GP or A&E doctor who can take a broad approach to whichever disease walks through the door on a particular day (**Figure 4.4**). This is a very gradual process which is already well under way, but I want you to start becoming more conscious of it from now on and incorporating it into your studies, right from the start of your penultimate year all the way to finals. This will

**Box 4.3**

**Seven clinically focused questions to ask yourself when learning about any disease:**

1. How would someone with this condition present?
2. How would I take a history from them?
3. Which examinations would I do and what would I expect to find?
4. What tests would I order and what results would I expect?
5. How would I explain the underlying anatomy and physiology to the patient in plain English?
6. How would I manage this condition?
7. What would I tell the patient about the next steps?

TOP TIP

There are many high-yield topics which start to appear in both OSCEs *and* written exams – therefore it makes no sense to treat your academic knowledge and clinical/communication skills as separate entities. Start taking a broad, 360° view of these conditions so that you are ready to tackle them in absolutely any forum or situation.

help you become more time-efficient, and will make life much easier when preparing for OSCEs. Because whether you like it or not, this change is already being forced upon you by your medical school making OSCE stations increasingly complex each year (and, to be fair to them, more representative of real-world practice). You risk getting a nasty surprise if you're not ready for this.

There are several ways you can accelerate this process, but the key is to start deliberately fusing your clinical and communication skills with your academic study instead of treating them as separate entities. Let's say you're learning about a new disease in your SDL time: in previous years you might have watched an online tutorial, written out a Dr Deac Pimp, tried a bunch of practice questions and made flashcards summarising the key points. From now on, you can go even further by

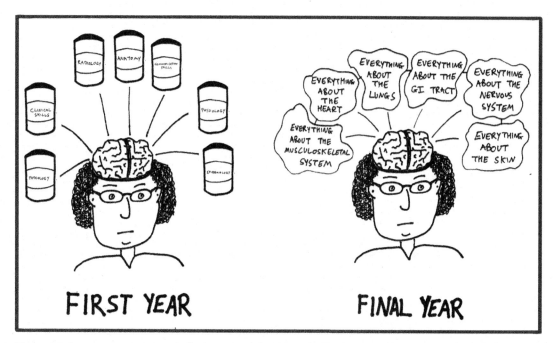

**Figure 4.4: As you progress towards final year, you should gradually start to integrate different subjects which were initially taught separately.** Move away from arbitrary silos in your brain to more fluid, interconnecting ideas focusing on the clinical issue at hand, rather than the order in which things were taught.

asking yourself the seven questions in **Box 4.3**, to get your brain in the zone of simultaneously thinking about OSCEs. And conversely, any time you practise clinical and communication skills with your friends, don't just run through tons of different histories and examinations: **do one then stop**, get your whiteboard pens out and have a proper good brainstorm of everything you know about that condition. Make sure everyone is comfortable with the key facts and feels they could recall them under

**Table 4.1: High-yield specialty topics that regularly come up in both OSCEs and written exams.** These underscore the need to start integrating your academic knowledge with your clinical and communication skills, because you will be examined on all of these different aspects

| Neurology | <ul><li>Migraine</li><li>Giant cell arteritis</li><li>Stroke and TIA</li><li>Epilepsy</li><li>Parkinson's</li><li>Multiple sclerosis</li><li>Dementia and delirium</li><li>Peripheral neuropathy</li><li>Bell's palsy</li><li>Myasthenia gravis</li></ul> |
|---|---|
| Psychiatry | <ul><li>Depression</li><li>Anxiety</li><li>Schizophrenia and psychosis</li><li>Bipolar disorder</li><li>Self-harm and suicidal ideation</li><li>Alcohol and drug misuse</li><li>Overdose</li><li>Sections of the Mental Health Act</li></ul> |
| Paediatrics | <ul><li>Non-accidental injury/safeguarding</li><li>Childhood infections</li><li>Febrile convulsions</li><li>Developmental delay</li><li>Faltering growth</li><li>Neonatal jaundice</li><li>Asthma/wheeze</li></ul> |

**Table 4.1:** *Continued*

| Obstetrics and gynaecology | • Pre-eclampsia |
| --- | --- |
| | • Gestational diabetes |
| | • Antenatal screening |
| | • Ectopic pregnancy |
| | • Miscarriage |
| | • Infertility |
| | • Cervical, ovarian and endometrial cancers |
| | • Polycystic ovarian syndrome |
| | • Endometriosis |
| | • Menstrual disorders and menopause |
| | • STIs and pelvic inflammatory disease |
| | • Contraception |
| | • Stress and urge urinary incontinence |
| | • Prolapse |

the pressure of an OSCE station before moving on to the next history or examination. This will make your practice sessions slower at first, but they will be much more valuable in the longer term. I really cannot stress this highly enough! Hopefully you are convinced, but **Table 4.1** has specific examples in case you need more persuading!

## 4.2.5 Group diseases by presenting complaint

Another useful way to develop your thinking in preparation for finals is to pick a common presenting complaint, then work out all the various conditions that could cause it and what steps would be required in the workup to establish a diagnosis. This reflects how real patients present – with a set of symptoms, not a diagnosis stuck to their forehead – so it's helpful to ensure you can come up with a wide range of possible explanations and know how you would go about differentiating between them.

This exercise is a method of flip reversing – a technique discussed in **Section 1.13**, whereby you approach the same piece of knowledge from different angles to ensure you really know it properly. For example, if I told you a patient had diabetes and asked for the main complications, you would probably suggest retinopathy. But if I told you that a patient presents with gradual loss of vision, would you **always** remember to suggest diabetes as one of the potential causes? In your first year, I suspect the answer would be no. By finals, the answer needs to be yes. That's where this exercise should help.

Another benefit to this approach is that once you start grouping conditions by their presenting complaint, you can ask yourself: "Realistically, which of these could appear in a finals OSCE station?" You will quickly realise that there are surprisingly few main presenting complaints! This is in contrast to the number of diagnoses you are expected to know about, which run to the hundreds if not thousands. Take respiratory medicine, for example: if you think about it, there are just four major presenting complaints: shortness of breath, cough, sputum production and haemoptysis. Cardiology also has four: chest pain, shortness of breath, palpitations and syncope. Neurology? Definitely more, but I still count only seven: headache, loss of consciousness, abnormal movements, weakness, altered sensation, altered cognition and altered speech. See **Table 4.2** for more.

**Table 4.2: The major presenting complaints for some of the specialties you will encounter in your penultimate year.** (Please note this is a simplification: of course there are additional presentations and symptoms that might arise, but these are the most common things that are likely to crop up in finals.)

| Specialty | Major presenting complaints |
|---|---|
| Gynaecology | • Heavy, light, absent or irregular menstrual bleeding<br>• Intermenstrual or post-coital bleeding<br>• Pelvic pain<br>• Abnormal vaginal discharge<br>• Subfertility<br>• Incontinence<br>• Prolapse |
| Paediatrics | • Jaundice<br>• Faltering growth<br>• Developmental delay<br>• Seizures<br>• Rash<br>• Unexplained injury<br>• Abdominal pain<br>• Vomiting or reflux<br>• Wheeze or difficulty breathing |

**Table 4.2:** *Continued*

| ENT | • Epistaxis<br>• Hearing loss<br>• Dizziness<br>• Tinnitus<br>• Dysphonia |
|---|---|
| GI surgery | • PR bleeding or haematemesis<br>• Change in bowel habit<br>• Vomiting<br>• Abdominal pain<br>• Difficulty swallowing<br>• Lumps<br>• Jaundice<br>• Weight loss |
| Ophthalmology | • Red eye<br>• Painful/itchy eye<br>• Gradual loss of vision<br>• Sudden loss of vision |
| Breast surgery | • Breast lump<br>• Breast pain<br>• Nipple discharge<br>• Skin changes |
| Rheumatology | • Painful joints<br>• Stiff joints<br>• Swollen joints |
| Urology | • Testicular pain<br>• Testicular lump<br>• Haematuria<br>• Lower urinary tract symptoms |

I found this approach comforting, as it makes everything feel much smaller and more manageable than when you are looking at enormous lists of diagnoses! In a paediatrics history OSCE station, for example, you know it's going to be one of these nine presenting complaints, so you better make damn sure you've practised them all and are confident at turning that presenting complaint into a diagnosis and management plan. Similarly, you'd be mad to head into an ENT station without knowing how to work up epistaxis, hearing loss, dizziness, tinnitus and dysphonia. So find some good OSCE scenarios where these are the presenting complaints, and practise, practise, practise!

## 4.2.6 Think forwards and backwards

If that approach appeals to you, you can also try working through the following exercise on paper by yourself, or on the whiteboard with friends:

- Pick a common presenting complaint (PC)
- Brainstorm all the possible diagnoses, grouped by body system
- Write out these subheadings: history, examination and investigations
- Pick a diagnosis and try to fill in the blank steps that carry you forwards from a presenting complaint to a diagnosis
- You only need to list the **major** positive findings or results, not every single thing
- Then cover it up and make sure you can also work in the reverse direction: backwards from the diagnosis to the presenting complaint.

Like so:

**Working forwards:**

PC  →  History  →  Examination  →  Investigations  →  Diagnosis

**Working backwards:**

Diagnosis  →  Investigations  →  Examination  →  History  →  PC

See **Figure 4.5** and **Table 4.3** for a worked example, using loss of consciousness as a presenting complaint and aortic stenosis as a diagnosis. This exercise is superb revision because it's covering you both for OSCEs, where you tend to start with a presenting complaint and try to work out the diagnosis, and written exams where you might be given any bit of the above information and asked to fill in any of the blanks. All that's missing is management, which is not part of this exercise but you will of course need to cover it as well.

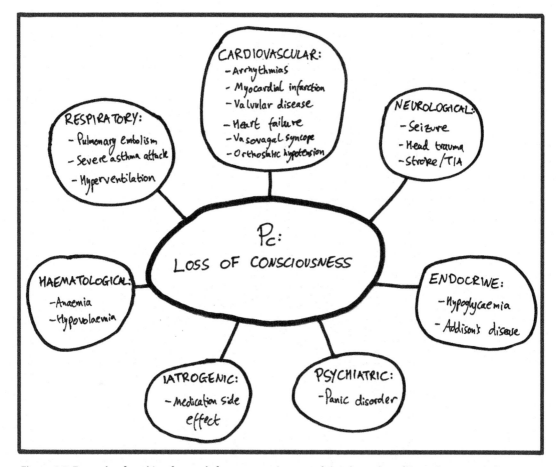

**Figure 4.5: Example of working forwards from presenting complaint through to diagnosis: part one.** Start by choosing a common or important presenting complaint, in this case loss of consciousness, and brainstorming all the possible diagnoses, grouped by body system. Then pick one diagnosis and continue the exercise as per *Table 4.3*.

**Table 4.3: Example of working forwards from presenting complaint through to diagnosis: part two.** Once you've picked a diagnosis, start with the middle three columns blank then try to fill them in from memory as a revision exercise. Then flip it around and work backwards from diagnosis to presenting complaint, filling in the boxes again. Repeat the whole exercise with a different diagnosis.[1]

| PC | History | Examination | Investigations | Diagnosis |
|---|---|---|---|---|
| Loss of consciousness | • Transient episode, recovered afterwards<br><br>• May be accompanied by chest pain, SOB and signs of heart failure<br><br>• Symptoms triggered by exertion, relieved by rest<br><br>• No neurological features | • Systolic murmur heard loudest at right upper sternal edge, radiating to carotids, augmented by leaning forwards<br><br>• Bibasal crepitations and ankle oedema (if accompanied by heart failure) | • Echo (definitive test): shows high flow gradient across valve, reduced valve area with impaired cusp opening, LV hypertrophy<br><br>• CXR: calcified aortic valve $\pm$ cardiomegaly<br><br>• ECG: non-diagnostic but may show LVH<br><br>• Bloods: BNP elevated if coexisting heart failure | Aortic stenosis |

### 4.2.7 Summary

In this section, we have looked at some techniques and ideas to carry you through your second clinical year and start preparing you for finals. The key points are:

- Bring together all the techniques you have used so far and focus on the ones that work best for you.
- Maintain efficiency with your studies so you can keep making time for yourself and avoid burnout at this crucial stage.
- Blitz any new specialty in three phases: reconnaissance, all-out assault and surveying the aftermath.
- Grab extra learning opportunities on offer, particularly in the specialties. These can be memorable and inspiring.
- Appreciate that there isn't much difference between the level of knowledge required for exams at the end of this year and finals.
- Integrate your academic studies with your clinical and communication skills as much as possible.
- Try new exercises such as grouping diseases by their presenting complaint then figuring out all the steps required to make a diagnosis, and vice versa.

# 4.3 Resources

By this stage, you're into your third, fourth or even fifth year of medical school and will know exactly which resources work well for you and which don't. Hopefully you've tried a broad range of different approaches and have got your 'go-to' books, apps and websites which you feel comfortable using. Still, it's never too late to try new things, and it is well worth re-appraising your resources and keeping an open mind for the year ahead.

This is particularly important as you venture into new specialties which you've not covered before: each has its own world of information ready for you to discover, so be prepared to go down the rabbit hole at least at the start of each new placement. This is also a good time to take stock and reflect on how last year went: did you spend too long on online question banks and not enough time covering the basics from books? Did you use flashcards so much you got sick of them? This year provides a blank slate to reset, refresh and try to get the balance right.

## 4.3.1 Books and websites

If you're in the market for a separate book for each specialty, check out series like **Pocket Tutor**, **Pocket Essentials** and the **Oxford Handbooks** for something small to carry around on placements. For larger books to use at home or in the library, check out **Table 4.4** for the major texts in each specialty. And of course remember those great series from **Table 2.6**, and MCQ books like **Get Ahead** and **Oxford Assess and Progress**.

Rather than going deep into every specialty, many people prefer to get one small pocket-sized book which covers a load of them in one go. The **Oxford Handbook of Clinical Specialties** does this very nicely and is, to my knowledge, the only small book that covers psychiatry, paediatrics and O&G in a single volume.

This is also a good year to start using clinical scenario/case study books in which you work through individual case studies in more detail than MCQs, answering multiple questions along the way as the case unfolds. **Clinical Cases Uncovered**, **100 Cases**, **Case Files**, **Oxford Case Histories** and **Core Clinical Cases** are all great examples of this.

Table 4.4: Overview of handy resources for clinical specialties

| Specialty | Books | Websites |
|---|---|---|
| **Paediatrics** | • *Illustrated Textbook of Paediatrics*<br>• *Crash Course Paediatrics*<br>• *The Unofficial Guide to Paediatrics* | • Royal College of Paediatrics and Child Health: www.rcpch.ac.uk/resources<br>• Don't Forget the Bubbles: http://dontforgetthebubbles.com |
| **Obstetrics and gynaecology** | • *Essential Obstetrics and Gynaecology*<br>• *Obstetrics and Gynaecology*<br>• *Obstetrics by Ten Teachers* | • Royal College of Obstetricians and Gynaecologists: www.rcog.org.uk/en/guidelines-research-services/ |
| **Psychiatry** | • *Psychiatry: a clinical handbook*<br>• *Textbook of Psychiatry*<br>• *Psychiatry PRN: principles, reality, next steps* | • Royal College of Psychiatrists' Psychiatry in Practice series: http://psychiatryinpractice.rcpsych.ac.uk |
| **Neurology** | • *Neurology: an illustrated colour text*<br>• *Neurological Examination Made Easy*<br>• *Neurology and Neurosurgery Illustrated* | • Ebrain. Includes practice questions: www.ebrain.net<br>• Association of British Neurologists: www.theabn.org/resources/ |

## 4.3.2 Guidelines

Your exposure to guidelines so far has probably been limited to other people telling you what's in them. In lectures about hypertension, for example, you were almost certainly given the NICE algorithm for selecting antihypertensive drugs, which you faithfully learned from the slides without ever going back to the original source. Likewise algorithms for the management of asthma, COPD, diabetes and many more.

Taking that information at face value has been fine so far, but now is probably the time to start going a little deeper by looking into clinical guidelines for yourself. This advice comes with a health warning: there is variation in the quality of guidelines, and at their worst they can be long, boring and confusing to read. But at their best they provide a great overview of a topic, with snappy up-to-date recommendations and clear advice on how to approach different situations. All doctors use guidelines in some form or another, so you will need to get used to them sooner or later. As a medical student I wouldn't spend **ages** on them, but definitely take a look and extract the key points, particularly when it comes to algorithms and pathways for diagnosis and treatment.

Start with NICE – these guidelines are the gold standard for the UK and much of the world – and the Clinical Knowledge Summaries that accompany each guideline. Be guided by your placements as to which ones to look at: in paediatrics, for example, you'll realise that the NICE guideline on 'Fever in under 5s' is extremely high yield, and it would be an error not to spend some time looking at it. Medical colleges and associations are also a great source of guidelines: in your O&G block, for example, you'll almost certainly be pointed towards guidelines from the Royal College of Obstetricians and Gynaecologists. Your local hospital or NHS Trust will also have its own guidelines which the junior doctors can show you.

If you still want more, there are various online portals for accessing an enormous array of clinical guidelines: try Evidence Search from NICE (www.evidence.nhs.uk), www.guidelines.co.uk, the Guidelines International Network (www.g-i-n.net) and www.guidelinecentral.com (this has an app too). You can also look on PubMed (www.pubmed.com) by filtering for guidelines within the advanced search function.

## 4.3.3 Journals

Similar to guidelines, I've steered clear of journals as a learning resource until now because they're not ideally suited to the early years of medical school. Journal articles can be dry and complex, requiring a lot of background knowledge to make any sense of. They also tend to focus on new developments at the cutting edge, which is of limited use to students who are still learning the fundamentals. I suspect most medical students avoid journals unless they are researching an essay or presentation, or have been told to look up a particular article. I certainly didn't use them much in the early years.

Nonetheless, journals are probably the number one medium by which doctors keep up to date with their specialty, and one of the main forums for discussion and debate (conferences are the other, but as a student you won't get much chance to go to these). Even as an FY1, you will probably have to attend and present at journal clubs – small meetings where you discuss and critique a journal paper – and might even get a chance to publish a paper of your own. So at some point you will have to engage with journals, and now is a reasonable time to at least dip your toe in the water!

You may have already started with the **BMJ**'s student-friendly articles, which are less intimidating than the grown-up journals to begin with. If you do want to move up the food chain though, you'll probably find it best to stick to the major general medical journals such as the **New England Journal of Medicine, JAMA, The Lancet** and the **BMJ**. These are the top dogs where the most prestigious research gets published and their articles tend to be very high-impact and relatively readable. They also have nice websites with up-to-date features like interactive image galleries, podcasts and videos – all of which makes for a far more enjoyable reading experience than some of the smaller journals!

Research papers, editorials, case reports and opinion pieces can all be interesting for your general knowledge, but be aware that they are unlikely to help you in your exams. Review articles, on the other hand, can provide a great overview of a subject and are often pitched at a reasonable level for medical students approaching final year. Since 2017 the **NEJM**, for example, has published reviews entitled Psychotic Disorders, Multiple Sclerosis and Hearing Loss in Adults, all of which are important high-yield topics for you to know about for finals. Search by article type to find these, either on PubMed or the journals' own sites, for example: www.nejm.org/medical-articles/review-article. Just ensure you choose your articles carefully and be wary about going too niche: the same link also offers reviews on Chimeric Antigen Receptor Therapy, Langerhans-Cell Histiocytosis and Mapping Symptoms to Brain Networks with the Human Connectome – topics which are about as useful to you right now as a chocolate teapot (no offence to the authors). You have been warned!

There are some great review articles to be found in the big four general medical journals: the *BMJ*, *The Lancet*, *NEJM* and *JAMA*. Check them out, but don't stray too far off-piste into stuff you really don't need to know about for finals!

TOP TIP

# 4.4 Pharmacology level II

Remember how in **Chapter 3** we talked about the importance of putting some proper effort into learning pharmacology? No? You've written it out of your memory already??

Well the good news is you've still got some time on your side to rectify the situation – but not much. Because in final year you will need to pass the Prescribing Safety Assessment (PSA) in order to graduate medical school and enter the Foundation Programme. We'll look at this in more detail in **Chapter 5**. But in the meantime, if you've not got on it yet, I would strongly encourage you to use your second clinical year to really get up to speed on pharmacology to avoid leaving it to the last minute when the PSA rolls around. Your future self will thank you!

If you have already built up a good knowledge of drugs and prescribing – in which case I salute you – then this is a good year to keep reinforcing and consolidating your knowledge. You will inevitably cover plenty of pharmacology as part of your placements, particularly on specialties when you are learning the management of a whole range of new conditions. But it's still worth treating it as a subject in its own right to ensure you keep developing your pattern recognition for answering pharmacology-focused exam questions. Here are some ways you can do that, with the PSA in mind:

- Blitz the pharmacology section of your favourite online question bank or the MCQs in clinical pharmacology books (**Table 3.2**). These are useful for boosting your rapid recall, as you will quickly start to spot recurring themes and questions which come up very regularly.

- Start working through extended prescribing scenarios from books such as **Prescribing Scenarios at a Glance** and **The Unofficial Guide to Prescribing**. These are great practice for the longer sections of the PSA and for life as an FY1.

- Keep looking at drug charts and testing yourself on the key facts about every drug. You should still be comfortable with paper drug charts, even if your hospital is fully electronic, because these come up in exams.

- Get quicker at looking things up in the **BNF** app or online. This is a useful skill as you will need to navigate it rapidly during the PSA.

- Start learning dosages for the most commonly prescribed drugs, as well as advice given to patients such as how and when to take them (we previously focused just on indications, mechanism of action, side-effects, warnings and interactions).

- Keep OSCEs in mind when studying pharmacology: medication-related stations come up very commonly from now on, so you should be comfortable explaining the pros and cons of particular medications using plain English that even your nan could understand.

- Spend some extra time studying tricky-to-prescribe drugs with potential for harm, notably insulin, opioids, steroids, anticoagulants, antibiotics, antidepressants and antipsychotics. These are high yield and come up a lot in exam questions.

- Another high-yield topic is prescribing restrictions for the four main 'specific patient groups' (that's how they're described in the **BNF**): pregnancy, breastfeeding, renal impairment and hepatic impairment. Ideally you should know off by heart the main drugs to avoid or dose-reduce in each of these groups.

- Get to grips with fluid prescribing (**Box 4.4**).

**Box 4.4**

> **Your second clinical year is a good time to start getting your head around fluid prescribing**
>
> I always found this very confusing as a student but I realise now that it seemed a lot worse than it really is. Here are three things to help demystify the topic:
> 1. There are only three fluids you will regularly prescribe as an FY1 and therefore need to know about for finals: 0.9% NaCl, Hartmann's and 5% dextrose. The others are just background noise.
> 2. Stick to adults – fluid prescribing for kids is too specialist for medical students.
> 3. Check out the NICE IV fluid algorithm: it looks complex at first but is actually extremely helpful. It's broken down into four sections and you can basically ignore the fourth one (replacement and redistribution) for now until you get more confident. So all you really need to know for this year is fluid status assessment (algorithm 1), fluid resuscitation (algorithm 2) and routine maintenance (algorithm 3). Once you realise that, it all feels a *lot* more manageable!
> www.nice.org.uk/guidance/cg174/resources/intravenous-fluid-therapy-in-adults-in-hospital-algorithm-poster-set-191627821

# 4.5 Clinical skills, communication skills and OSCEs: level III

In **Chapter 2** we looked at general principles for history taking and examination such as structured frameworks, working anatomically, sticking to the script and practising on your friends. Then in **Chapter 3** we moved things forward by introducing real patients, discussed ways to develop your thinking process and history-taking skills and looked at how to evolve your practice sessions with your friends. Believe me, you've already come a long way in this short space of time: **you are starting to look, think and act like a doctor**, even if you don't feel like one yet!

For your second clinical year, we'll take things up a few more notches to get you ready for your finals. As we noted in **Section 4.2.3**, there really isn't much gap between what you're expected to know at the end of penultimate year and the end of final year. For that reason, this will be our last dip into the world of clinical and communication skills together: I'll give you all the hints and tricks I've got left in my locker, so you can start developing yourself into the finished product at your own pace.

> Don't put off learning new clinical and communication techniques until next year: challenge yourself to reach your peak by the end of **this** year, then use final year to practise, reinforce and consolidate those existing skills.

**TOP TIP**

## 4.5.1 Add specialty histories to your repertoire

You already learned the generic template for any medical history way back in your preclinical years: presenting complaint, history of the presenting complaint, past medical and surgical history, medication history, family history and social history. Then in the last chapter we looked at how to start customising that template according to the situation you are facing; for example, asking about smoking early in a chest pain history, or looking for VTE risk factors in someone with sudden-onset shortness of breath.

Now you've got a new challenge as you discover the clinical specialties: you'll realise they each have their own template for history taking, which takes you back to the drawing board to learn them from scratch. These templates are rigid, proscriptive and taken very seriously by their practitioners, who will expect you to know them properly.

**It's like each specialty has its own secret handshake which you need to learn in order to fit in. Ask about immunisations in a paediatric history, for example, and you'll get a nod and a knowing smile. Forget to ask about alcohol and drugs in a psychiatric history, and you've committed a faux pas so serious that no psychiatrist will ever send you a Christmas card again.**

**KEY POINT**

Psychiatry, paediatrics and obstetrics and gynaecology each have their own structures for history taking. You'll need to go back to the drawing board and learn these from scratch.

Check out **Box 4.5** for the basic templates for history taking in paediatrics, O&G and psychiatry. As ever in medicine, there is loads of variation and my templates may differ from yours: if in doubt, default back to what your med school taught you.

**Box 4.5**

### Templates for specialty histories

You'll need to learn these off by heart and quickly get up to speed with using them.

**Paediatric history**
- Basics: who is the child and who is the history taken from?
- Presenting complaint
- History of presenting complaint
- Past medical history
- Birth history
- Developmental history
- Feeding history
- Immunisation history
- Medication history
- Social history

**Obstetric history**
- Basics: gestational age, gravidity, parity and maternal age
- Presenting complaint
- History of presenting complaint
- History of the current pregnancy
- Past obstetric history
- Gynaecological history
- Past medical and surgical history
- Medication and contraception history
- Family history
- Social history

**Box 4.5** *continued*

**Gynaecological history**
- Basics: gravidity, parity and date of last menstrual period
- Presenting complaint
- History of presenting complaint
- Menstrual history
- Contraception
- Cervical screening
- Past gynaecological history
- Past medical and surgical history
- Obstetric history
- Medication history
- Family history
- Social history

**Psychiatric history**
- Presenting complaint
- History of presenting complaint
- Family history
- Past psychiatric history
- Past medical and surgical history
- Alcohol and drug use
- Medication history
- Forensic history
- Personal history, including early development, education, occupation and sexual history
- Pre-morbid personality

These templates are just the basic skeletons: there is absolutely loads of detail to flesh out on top, in particular the specific symptoms you are looking for in each type of history. It takes a lot of hard work and practice to get good at these histories, and you are really up against it in terms of time. You had two or three years to practise and perfect the basic medical history; now you've got just five or six weeks to learn each of these new ones, on top of all the other material you need to cover in specialty placements.

**Specialty histories are the very definition of high yield: virtually guaranteed to come up in OSCEs. There's no way around them except to learn the structures and practise, practise, practise.**

The only solution is to take these histories very seriously and start practising them as early and as regularly as you can. Consider yourself on an accelerated programme: you will need to learn the structure of the history inside out, then almost immediately work out how to customise it, then perfect the whole shebang as quickly as you can. Put history taking at the top of your list of things to study in each specialty, practise with as many real patients as you can and run through scenarios with your friends whenever you get the chance. See **Table 3.2** for a reminder of some OSCE resources for finals level – these will really prove invaluable at this stage.

## 4.5.2 **Present cases more effectively**

In the last chapter, I suggested presenting cases to your seniors wherever possible and getting feedback on your presentations. A year later, you've hopefully had a good go at doing this.

For the next stage, let's focus on ways to improve your case presentations because this is an important skill which you really don't get much teaching on at medical school. Perhaps because of this, plus the fact that it's not formally assessed, students often see case presentations as a tedious chore you need to perform just to get your CBDs and mini-CEXs signed off. This is a shame because it's a huge part of being a junior doctor – as an FY1 I am constantly presenting patients to the medical registrar in A&E, or to the consultant on ward rounds – so it's definitely worth putting in some effort to boost your confidence and ability early on. Good presentations are vital for patient care as they enable colleagues to quickly get to grips with the most important and relevant aspects of a case in a short space of time, allowing them to make decisions and provide further expertise and input.

I wanted you to have a proper go at presenting cases under your own steam before providing any pointers. It's difficult when you first start, right? What were the main issues you faced? Having been through this process, **Box 4.6** shows what I would have said at the end of my first clinical year.:

If you recognise any of these feelings then don't beat yourself up about it because I can assure you, with the benefit of hindsight, that these are natural and unavoidable steps which we all must go through in order to improve. Patient presentation is a skill that is learned informally through trial and error, getting feedback and making small changes one tweak at a time. There is also a huge amount of knowledge and experience required to know exactly what's relevant and you are still acquiring both of these, so don't be hard on yourself. Keep going and you **will** get there, I promise!

**Common struggles students face when presenting patients to a senior**

Box 4.6

- My presentations are too long and waffly.
- I don't know yet what information is most relevant, so I err on the side of giving too much rather than too little.
- I follow the structure of a standard medical history when presenting, yet my listener often seems to get bored and lose interest.
- I tend to zoom in on a particular diagnosis without properly excluding all the differentials.
- I must have asked the patient a hundred questions – but sod's law dictates the listener *still* thinks of something I didn't cover.
- My management plans are sketchy at best.
- The listener often cuts me off before I have finished, which is demoralising when I've done a great clerking.

You have now taken the first step on the road to better case presentations, which is to recognise that this is actually a skill in its own right which can be improved through effort and practice. Hopefully your medical school will at least provide **some** guidance, but if not there are helpful tutorials on YouTube: for starters, check out the University of Calgary's **Signpost Method**, Rahul Patwari's **Presenting Patients** and EM in 5's **Patient Presentations**.[2]

I've also developed my own top 13 suggestions based on my experiences – good and bad – and the feedback I received. These are for use on clinical placements when presenting to real doctors, as opposed to in an artificial OSCE or academic setting.

1. **Think carefully before you start about what you're going to say.** Sometimes we get so preoccupied with finding someone to listen to our presentation that we forget to plan the actual thing! Take five minutes to think it through beforehand – don't just start spewing out information without mentally rehearsing it.

2. **Always have a list of differentials and a management plan.** These are often an afterthought when students first start presenting cases, but for a doctor listening to your presentation these are what the entire exercise is about. They want to see that you're progressing from a preclinical student who is focused on the **process** of information gathering to a soon-to-be-doctor who is focused on what to **actually do** with that information.

---

2 Signpost Method: www.youtube.com/watch?v=Mew2wzpuhTs
  Presenting Patients: www.youtube.com/watch?v=4kgkCgLg1xE
  Patient Presentations: www.youtube.com/watch?v=isM2MJdRjyE

3.  **Keep it short.** Doctors are only humans with limited attention spans and – yes, it's true – they will quickly glaze over if they find your presentation boring (*Figure 4.6*). Try to keep it to two minutes maximum unless specifically invited to go into more depth. Sure, the patient gave you loads more info, but you don't need to include it all.

4.  **Signpost at the start.** Set the listener's expectations by briefly telling them what you've done and what you intend to cover in your presentation. For example: *"I've taken a history and examined Mrs Nguyen in bed 8, would you mind if I presented a short summary of the case along with my differentials and management plan?"* If you think there is urgency then say so straight away – don't talk for 10 minutes before concluding that the patient is having a STEMI.

5.  **Be engaging.** Stand up straight, speak clearly and make eye contact. Above all, appear interested in what you're saying – if you seem bored, there's no hope for the listener!

6.  **Consider your audience.** A psychiatrist might care about a patient's job, hobbies and sex life; a cardiothoracic surgeon probably won't. Give the listener what they want by focusing on the details most relevant to the specialty and situation at hand.

7.  **Have a snappy opening line to grab the listener's attention.** Focus on the presenting complaint and key symptoms, but include just enough relevant background to start their brain whirring. Always include age and gender. For example: *Mr Ali is a 53-year-old smoker with type 2 diabetes who has presented to A&E with a 5-hour history of central constricting chest pain radiating to his neck with associated sweating and nausea.* Note the inclusion of smoker and type 2 diabetes right at the start because they are extremely relevant to the presenting complaint.[3]

8.  **Avoid long lists of symptoms and signs.** Provide only the most relevant positives and negatives from the history and examination. You are trying to build a clear narrative, so focus on things that support your differentials rather than muddying the waters by listing absolutely everything you discussed with the patient.

---

3 Alternatively you can state their occupation: *"Mr Ali is a 53-year-old teacher who presents with ..."*. I picked this up from a surgeon who had one of the best bedside manners I've ever encountered. He argued that occupation demonstrates immediately that you have spent time talking to the patient and see them as a human being. And of course, some jobs are risk factors for diseases, which is clinically relevant. I love this idea – I tend to prioritise urgent clinical information such as *smoker with type 2 diabetes* – but if there is nothing urgent I'll go with occupation.

9.  **Mix up the structure.** You don't need to trundle through each section of the history one after another – after exploring the presenting complaint you could just say *"He has a background of ..."* and then merge all the key parts of the past medical, medication, family and social histories into one. There are lots of options for an order, but one suggestion would be: Presenting complaint – Background – Examination – Differentials – Management.

10. **State diseases and drugs together.** This flows naturally and will save you a lot of words, for example: *"He has hypertension for which he takes lisinopril and amlodipine, and type 2 diabetes managed with metformin."*

11. **Show your working.** When presenting your differential diagnoses, pick no more than three and suggest why you think each one is/ isn't the diagnosis and what you would like to do to rule it in or out: *"Given the classical symptoms and the history of smoking and diabetes, I think this is most likely to be an acute coronary syndrome. I would like to get an ECG and serial troponins to differentiate between a STEMI, NSTEMI and unstable angina, plus routine bloods and a chest X-ray. Other differentials include acute pericarditis, which would be evident on the ECG, and pulmonary embolism, for which I would consider taking a D-dimer, calculating the Wells Score and ordering a CTPA if indicated from the history."*

12. **Approach management like an FY1:** keep your management plan to the basic steps that would be expected of a junior doctor, then know who to refer to. It's unrealistic to say you would do everything yourself! For example: *"I would stabilise the patient using an ABCDE approach and instigate initial management with aspirin, morphine, a nitrate, oxygen and clopidogrel or ticagrelor as per local ACS protocol. I would then refer urgently to cardiology for consideration of primary PCI."*

13. **Try to get some informal teaching off it:** presenting a case gives you an 'in' to starting a conversation with a doctor so it's a great opportunity to get some informal teaching. When you're finished presenting, ask for feedback then follow up with a few questions about aspects of the case you weren't sure about. Or ask to review the patient's investigation results and imaging together. More often than not they'll be happy to chat, once you've demonstrated your interest and enthusiasm.

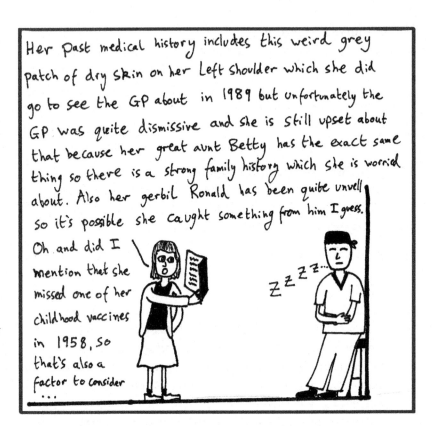

**Figure 4.6: Presenting cases to a senior can be very challenging at first, as it is hard to know how much information to include.** Try to keep your presentations short and concise without reading from notes, otherwise you risk putting your listener to sleep.

Always remember that however amazing your presentation, you will probably **still** receive feedback on things you could improve (hopefully you got some positive feedback as well!). I'm afraid this is just a fact of life – everyone has their own style of presenting patients and there is simply no correct way to do it. So at some point, once you feel your presentations have improved as far as you can take them, it is okay to politely accept the feedback then decide to ignore it. You can't please all the people all the time! And if a doctor really dumps on your presentation when you thought it had gone well, you can always try it again with someone else!

### 4.5.3 Customise your examinations

In clinical and communication skills level I, I stressed that you should perform examinations exactly as you were taught, following all the steps in the right order no matter how obscure they seem. Then for level II, we looked at how to get yourself quickly to the diagnosis then go back and tick the extra boxes to scoop up more marks. Now, for the final phase, level III, we will talk about how to customise your examinations and add some style and flair on top.

The main ways to do this are to adjust the order of your examination and add special tests **depending on the pathology you are faced with.** This is a natural progression from level II where we focused on working out the diagnosis as quickly as possible – now that you can recognise the diagnosis, level III is about exploring it in more depth to demonstrate that you **really** understand all aspects of that condition. It's no longer enough just to get the diagnosis then mic drop. Level III is also about demonstrating hypothesis testing (**Section 3.6.2**) – showing the examiner that you tested and excluded all the plausible alternatives before settling on your diagnosis.

You have more licence to customise your examinations now, so as soon as you have a suspected diagnosis in mind you should start to tailor your actions towards it. Here are seven ways you can do that:

> **Seven ways to customise your examination once you have a diagnosis in mind.**
> 1. Do the most relevant steps of the examination first.
> 2. Spend more time on relevant steps and less time on irrelevant steps.
> 3. Add in special tests or bring in useful bits of other examinations.
> 4. Try to actively exclude differential diagnoses.
> 5. Show insight to the condition and its complications (**Section 4.5.4**).
> 6. Only then go back and complete all the remaining, less relevant steps.
> 7. Know exactly what other tests you would need to complete your examination and why.

See **Table 4.5** for an example of how students at different stages of medical school might approach a neurological examination on a patient with Parkinson's disease. Abdominal examination is another which is easy to customise: if you are suspecting renal disease, for example, you should take time to look for fistulas and tunnelled lines, auscultate for renal bruits, ballot the kidneys, palpate the iliac fossae for transplanted kidneys, look for conjunctival pallor and inspect extra carefully for scars. If you spot a stoma, on the other hand, leave the renal stuff till later and focus on inspecting and describing the stoma and looking for clues to the underlying bowel disease: check for finger clubbing, oral ulcers and pyoderma gangrenosum to show you are thinking of inflammatory bowel disease, for example. You can apply these principles to any examination. See **Box 4.7** for more examples of how you can customise examinations to go above and beyond the standard template that every other student is using.

There are just a couple of small but important health warnings to add: first, you need to think about these extra steps and practise them **well in advance** so that anything you add in looks slick and confident (it's

**Table 4.5: Example of how students at different stages of medical school might perform a neurological examination on a patient with Parkinson's disease in an OSCE.** Please note that level III would be an extremely high level of performance, probably worthy of a distinction, so don't panic if you're not at that level yet! This is just to illustrate the progression through the years and give you a target to aim for.

| Level I: Preclinical years | Level II: Early clinical years | Level III: Finals |
|---|---|---|
| • Performs a full neurological examination, exactly as they would on any patient, following the standard structure of inspection, tone, power, coordination, sensation and reflexes<br><br>• Suggests Parkinson's disease as their top differential<br><br>• Throws in some other random neurological conditions just to cover their bases | • Begins a standard neurological examination but recognises early on that this is Parkinson's disease<br><br>• Focuses on assessing gait, tone and tremor, commenting in detail on these before finishing the rest of the examination<br><br>• Confidently states Parkinson's disease as their top differential<br><br>• Mentions Parkinson-plus conditions such as multiple system atrophy and progressive supranuclear palsy, as well as other causes of tremor such as essential and cerebellar tremor, but does not actively attempt to rule these in or out | • Almost immediately recognises Parkinson's disease and assesses the patient's gait, tone and tremor<br><br>• Also comments on speech and facial expression (hypophonia and hypomimia)<br><br>• Uses special tests to elicit cog-wheeling, bradykinesia and the glabellar reflex<br><br>• Assesses eye movements and postural reflexes to exclude the Parkinson-plus conditions, and tests for any coexisting cerebellar dysfunction<br><br>• Only then goes back to finish the rest of the standard neurological examination<br><br>• Confidently states that the patient has Parkinson's disease and comments on how advanced it is, using appropriate language and empathy<br><br>• Explains that their examination has so far excluded Parkinson-plus conditions; however, they would like to assess lying and standing blood pressure to fully rule out multisystem atrophy and formally assess cognition to rule out Lewy body dementia<br><br>• Specifies why essential and cerebellar tremor are less likely based on their examination findings<br><br>• Discusses ongoing management, avoidance of complications and psychosocial aspects of the disease |

extremely risky to try out new things for the first time in an OSCE!). This is where having the station titles in advance can really help (**Section 3.6.7**), as it gives you one last chance to consider all the possible permutations that might come up. Ideally, only bring in extra steps that you have witnessed doctors do in real life and have practised for yourself on real patients. If you are not sure you can pull it off then just stick to the basics: it's always better to do a routine examination to a high standard than to make a mess of going off-piste. And secondly, if you are customising your examination in an OSCE, it is sensible to state out loud what you are doing so that the examiner can follow. They aren't necessarily experts in that field so might not know the extra tests – make it clear that you aren't just making things up as you go along!

**Box 4.7**

---

**Examples of ways to customise your examinations to reach level III of clinical skills**

**Musculoskeletal examinations:** have some special tests up your sleeve to add in depending on the suspected pathology; e.g. if you suspect rotator cuff pathology in a shoulder exam, you could do the 'empty can test' and assess for painful arc. In a hand and wrist exam, do Phalen's and Tinel's tests if suspecting carpal tunnel syndrome or Finkelstein's test for de Quervain's tenosynovitis.

**Respiratory examination:** if you think the patient has COPD, assess for features of heart failure to demonstrate that you understand cor pulmonale is a potential complication. And state that you would like an arterial blood gas to assess for chronic respiratory failure and an FBC to assess for anaemia or polycythaemia.

**Abdominal exam on renal patient:** if the patient has an active fistula, assess their fluid status, check for confusion, asterixis and excoriations and state that you would like to check U&Es and an ECG. This shows you are considering acute dialysis-related complications such as fluid overload, uraemia and hyperkalaemia. In any renal patient, state you would like to check HbA1c and blood pressure, because diabetes and hypertension are the leading causes of end-stage renal failure.

**Peripheral vascular exam:** describe ulcers in detail and suggest whether the pathology is arterial or venous. If you suspect arterial, focus on palpating pulses and check for cyanosis and tar staining. If you suspect venous, focus on characterising skin changes, working out which part of the venous system is affected and looking for a saphena varix. Know about special tests like Buerger's, the tap and tourniquet tests, but be aware these aren't performed much nowadays.

### 4.5.4 Build up muscle memory and pattern recognition

You're now at the stage where you need to resemble a real doctor when you perform an examination or take a history. And I don't mean having bags under your eyes, being unable to work the computers or smelling faintly of the last patient's piss: I mean looking polished, professional and purposeful.

**The best way to *look* like you have done something before is – stop the presses – to have *actually* done it before. Hundreds of times. On real patients as well as your friends.**

**Box 4.8**

**Top tips for improving your pattern recognition and muscle memory in your second clinical year**

- Make the most of unstructured ward time instead of skiving off like in previous years.
- If there's nothing happening in your ward, head to others in search of interesting patients and signs. FY1s can usually point you in the right direction (our WhatsApp group is constantly pinging with 'Anyone got any patients for the medical students to examine?').
- In clinics, ask the consultant if there is a spare room where you can see some patients on your own before presenting the case to them. This can be scary but is an absolutely amazing way to learn. Not every consultant will be up for this, but if you find one who is, you should take the opportunity.
- Make an extra effort during paediatrics, psychiatry and O&G placements to take histories and perform examinations. These are crucial skills in their own right, and you only get a short window to practise them.
- GP and A&E placements are excellent opportunities for you to practise seeing new patients who have a completely unfiltered array of symptoms.
- Any time you examine a patient, challenge yourself to get faster without sacrificing accuracy.
- Focus more on getting to the right diagnosis, as compared to previous years where you placed more emphasis on the *process* of history taking and examination. If you did a nice examination but missed the key signs, go back and check them out.

So if you've somehow managed to get this far while barely laying hands on the general public, I'd suggest it's time for a rethink. Use this year to clerk and examine **as many patients as possible** in preparation for your finals. This will help you build up pattern recognition, muscle memory and make everything flow much more instinctively. The more clinical signs you see, the quicker you will recognise them next time. The more histories you take, the better you will get at extracting the key information.

This is particularly true for the specialties, where you need to bed in those new history templates as quickly as possible. You also need to **seriously** practise examining children during your paediatrics placements: they are a completely different species (trust me, I've got three of them at home) and interacting with them requires a whole new skill set (**Figure 4.7**). It will be **extremely** obvious to an OSCE examiner if you've never done it before! Ditto a gynaecologist watching you perform a bimanual palpation, an obstetrician watching you take an obstetric history or a psychiatrist watching you perform a mental state examination. They'll know if you're blagging it.

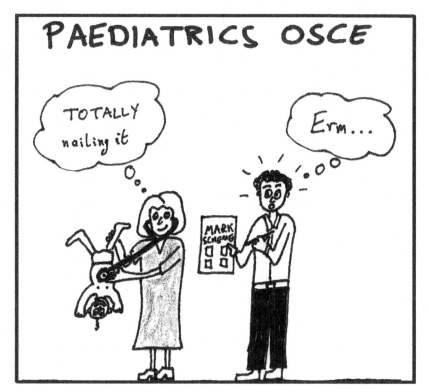

Figure 4.7: An OSCE station is a very bad setting to be examining children for the first time. Make sure you are comfortable, confident and have done it loads of times before on your placements.

## 4.5.5 Display and use insight

An important way to do well in OSCEs (and be a better doctor!) is to demonstrate insight to the patient and their disease, and show that you don't see them simply as some sort of zoo specimen. This can be easier said than done, particularly under pressure in OSCEs. But it's nonetheless something to aspire to, particularly as the patient/actor usually assigns you a score as part of the mark scheme so it is vital to keep them onside. Patients and actors have different values to examiners, and are **way** more interested in your bedside manner and choice of words than your recognition of clinical signs. My mum, for example, still vividly remembers an obstetrician presenting her to the medical students as an "elderly primigravida" (she was aged 30 at the time). All these years later she remains pissed off about it, and frankly I don't blame her!

**TOP TIP**

During your OSCE preparations, think about ways to display insight and compassion to the patient and their situation that go beyond mere signs and symptoms. Build these into your practice so that you get into this habit, and won't forget to do it under pressure on the day.

Hopefully you're polite, professional and courteous and would never make that sort of clanger! But nevertheless for OSCE finals we need to think about clever ways to link your observations, examination findings and background knowledge to the human face sitting in front of you, to appeal to the examiner and the patient *at the same time*. There are lots of ways you can do this: below are just four suggestions. You can use more than one in a single station. In each case, be sure to use your insight by *linking it* to your plan and next steps, even if you don't have time to do everything in the station:

1. **Consider the *severity* of their disease:** e.g. in an asthma station, make sure you take a proper look at any inhalers the patient has lying around. If they are on a SABA, medium-dose inhaled steroid and a LABA, for example, you know that they are on at least step 3 of the BTS/SIGN guidelines algorithm for asthma management. State this for the examiner's benefit, but be sure to put it into plain English too: *"Mr Hamilton's inhalers suggest he has had a difficult time getting his asthma under control and has unfortunately required several changes to his medications."*

   → **Link it to your plan:** *"If we had more time in this station, I would like to review Mr Hamilton's inhaler technique and his asthma action* plan to make sure he knows what to do in the event of his breathing becoming more difficult. If he still experiences symptoms on his current inhalers, I'd consider adding a fourth drug such as a leukotriene receptor antagonist and referring to an asthma specialist for further advice."

2. **Consider the *impact* on the patient:** e.g. in a hand and wrist examination, if the patient has rheumatoid arthritis, make sure to carry out a functional assessment, such as by asking them to do up a button, pick up a coin or write their name. Comment on the findings with appropriate empathy: *"Mrs Lucas is unfortunately having difficulty picking up small objects and holding a pen, suggesting her arthritis could be really affecting her day-to-day life."*

   → **Link it to your plan:** *"If we had more time, I'd like to explore in more detail the impact of Mrs Lucas' arthritis on her home and work life and consider referring to physiotherapy and occupational therapy for extra advice and support. I'd also like to take a more detailed medication history, and ensure she is under a rheumatologist so she can access disease-modifying therapies which will prevent her joints from deteriorating further."*

3. **Take a broad, *holistic* view:** e.g. after taking a history from someone with depression, consider biological, psychological and social aspects of their condition: *"Mr Vazquez has a strong family history of depression, which may have predisposed him to the condition. He also displays negative thinking patterns such as rumination and inappropriate guilt, compounded by his recent divorce and fear that he might lose his job due to sickness absences."*

   → **Link it to your plan:** *"I'd like to refer Mr Vazquez for cognitive behavioural therapy to address some of his negative thinking patterns and consider starting him on an antidepressant such as an SSRI. He might also benefit from a supported return to work, so I would direct him to sources of information such as the Fit for Work free advice line."*

4. **Anticipate *complications* of their condition:** e.g. if your patient has diabetes: *"It appears from the history and blood tests that Ms King has undiagnosed diabetes with poor blood sugar control. This places her at high risk of developing cardiovascular disease, particularly as she is a smoker with an unhealthy diet, and microvascular complications such as neuropathy, nephropathy and retinopathy."*

   → **Link it to your plan:** *"Ms King will need 3-monthly HbA1c checks in the short term, plus annual reviews of her feet, eyes, blood pressure, renal* *function and cholesterol as part of her routine diabetes care. I would also provide advice on exercise and healthy eating, and consider referring for smoking cessation support. Depending on her results, she may require antidiabetic medications, antihypertensives and/or a statin."*

**TOP TIP**

In any OSCE station, remember the patient's name, be polite and friendly and make eye contact when talking to them. Don't just pretend they've left the room when you're talking to the examiner: continue to use the appropriate language in front of them.

## 4.5.6 Develop your procedural skills

I have another confession to make: I never got fully confident with practical procedures at medical school. It wasn't for lack of trying: I did absolutely loads. And it wasn't lack of success either: I took blood, sited cannulas, got ABGs and inserted catheters – not always at the first attempt, and with a far from 100% success rate, but with many achieved nonetheless. But somehow the unsuccessful attempts haunted me and I irrationally fixated on them: I had caused the patient pain for no benefit, I looked silly in front of the FY1, I wasted equipment, and so on. I always tensed up as I headed to the bedside with my little tray of equipment, and would feel an immense sense of relief once I'd finished.

The truth is, I didn't get over this anxiety until around halfway through FY1. It was only when I started taking blood on an almost daily basis that I became comfortable with it. I must have done hundreds now and you know what? I'm actually good at it! I've had several patients compliment me on my technique (just the other day: "Ooooh you're good – I barely felt that!") and often manage to bleed patients where phlebotomists have failed. Last weekend I very delicately took blood from a patient with idiopathic thrombocytopenic purpura and a platelet count of 5 (very high risk for bleeding and bruising) while barely leaving a mark on her skin. I've still got some way to go on the other skills, but blood taking is finally in my comfort zone.

I'm telling you this not to show off, but to reassure those of you out there who are also struggling with these feelings that they are perfectly normal and probably much more common than you think. I thought I'd never get over my anxieties but I did in the end, and so can you. Some people are confident with procedures from day one and others never get there, but most of us are somewhere in the middle: it is only after a serious amount of practice that we get comfortable doing these fiddly, unpleasant and painful things to our fellow human beings. As a med student, you are probably not hitting the volumes required to get 100% confident yet, but believe me your time will come if you keep on practising. In the meantime, here are my top tips which will hopefully help you along the way (**Box 4.9**).

---

**Top tips for improving your procedural skills and confidence**

- Always double-check your equipment before you head to the bedside and take extra supplies in case you don't succeed first time. It's annoying for both you and the patient to have to go back and get more stuff.
- Don't rush: give veins a little time to swell up once the tourniquet is on, and choose your target carefully.
- Prepare properly by thinking about lighting, positioning and ensuring both you and the patient are comfortable.
- Remember to keep talking to the patient and reassuring them: it's usually much worse for them than for you.[4]
- Have all the equipment immediately to hand: it's a nightmare to get the needle in then realise you can't reach the blood bottles or gauze.
- Fix the vein firmly in place with your non-dominant hand, especially in older people. This step is easily missed, and calcified veins can bounce out of the needle's way.
- Insert needles using a confident forward motion. However tentative you feel, do not let that transmit to your hands by jabbing half-heartedly then pulling back.
- Don't panic if you don't immediately get flashback. Just keep the needle in, make small, careful adjustments and it will usually come soon enough.
- If you are struggling, find extra opportunities to practise under supervision, such as outpatient phlebotomy for bloods, ambulance handover for cannulation, A&E resus for ABGs and operating theatres, geriatrics or urology wards for catheters.

---

## 4.5.7 OSCEs: expect the unexpected

Back in the early years, OSCE stations tended to be clean and clear-cut. You had one, maybe two tasks to complete in the allocated time: usually straightforward examinations or histories, with perhaps some results or imaging thrown in towards the end. You presented your findings and

---

4 This isn't *always* the case: I recently had a patient tell me she absolutely loved having her blood taken and asked if it could be done daily. She was genuinely disappointed to be told she was being discharged and didn't need any more blood tests!

differentials, answered a few questions from the examiner and moved on to the next station. Job done.

As you head towards finals, however, things start to get messier. Now they have licence to throw almost anything at you, and will frequently do so – often giving you multiple different tasks in the same station (**Figure 4.8**). It might begin as an obstetrics history, move into interpretation of blood pressure and urine results to diagnose pre-eclampsia, then test your pharmacology knowledge and communication skills as the patient asks you loads of questions about labetalol. A psychiatry station can test your temperament and people skills when the patient becomes aggressive, then morph into ethics and law when they refuse treatment and you need to discuss sectioning under the Mental Health Act. A respiratory history points to a straightforward pneumonia, then the patient's observations deteriorate and you're suddenly into the acute management of sepsis using an ABCDE approach. I once had a lower limb neurology examination which progressed into telling the patient that they had poorly controlled diabetes and were at risk of needing their foot amputated. That's a lot of different skills being tested at once!

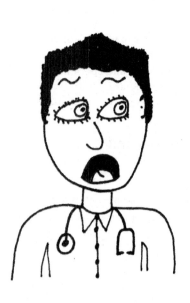

**Figure 4.8: OSCE stations become more complex and multifaceted as you progress through medical school.** Expect the unexpected and be prepared for changes of direction midway through.

FINAL YEAR OSCE:

STATION 5

Mr Musa has attended the GP today with a headache. Please take a history from him.

After 4 minutes, the examiner will hand you a recipe which you will need to cook using only your left hand and ingredients containing the letter q.

The buzzer will sound with 2 minutes to go: this is your cue to begin dancing a ceilidh whilst juggling packets of aspirin and spelling the word 'sphygmomanometer' out loud in a French accent.

In penultimate- and final-year OSCEs, expect the unexpected and be ready for just about anything. Stations can rapidly change tack midway through, forcing you to think on your feet and re-adjust.

**TOP TIP**

I can't tell you **exactly** what sort of things will come up at your medical school, so I hope you made friends in the years above who can give you some pointers! But **Box 4.10** contains some suggestions based on my experiences and those of my friends at other med schools. You should prepare for this by having a go at all of these skills in your practice sessions with friends, starting as soon as possible. No matter how confident you feel about them, you can always practise more to improve your style and choice of words. It is also helpful to start including multiple different tasks in your mock OSCE stations, so that you get used to pivoting midway through. You've got the knowledge and skills to boss this now – don't let them catch you out with their sneaky little tricks!

---

**Challenging types of OSCE station which classically come up in penultimate year and finals**

**Box 4.10**

Note that you may face multiple different tasks within the same station.

**Communication skills:**
- Breaking bad news
- Discussing DNAR orders
- Dealing with angry or aggressive patients
- Safeguarding
- Domestic abuse
- Drugs and alcohol
- Consent, capacity and confidentiality
- Explaining a diagnosis, medication, investigation or procedure
- Awareness of DVLA rules on driving with certain medical conditions
- Mental state examination.

**Clinical skills:**
- Management of an acutely unwell patient using an ABCDE approach
- Examining patients with multiple different signs
- Examining more than one body system
- Examinations that evolve and change midway through
- 'Intimate' examinations: breast, rectal, testicular or speculum
- Interpreting multiple investigations
- Prescribing drugs, fluids or both
- Setting up an intravenous infusion
- Trickier procedures such as catheterisation or suturing
- Demonstrating inhaler technique.

## 4.5.8 Summary

In this section, we have looked at tips to help you survive your second year of placements and take your clinical and communication skills up to the level required for final-year OSCEs. The key points are:

- There isn't much difference between the level expected of a penultimate year student versus a finals student, so try to aspire to finals level from now on.

- Learn the specialty histories (paediatrics, psychiatry and O&G) inside out: these are very high yield and extremely likely to come up in OSCEs.

- Work on improving your patient presentations: this is an essential skill for life as a doctor.

- Customise your examinations according to the patient and their pathology.

- Examine and clerk hundreds of real patients so you can recognise signs, look slick and get skilled at gathering information.

- Display insight to a patient's disease by considering its severity, potential complications, the impact on their life and taking a broader view than just the medical aspects.

- Incorporate those insights into your management plan to ensure you actually address the issues you have raised.

- Keep working on your procedural skills, and don't be disheartened if you are still finding it difficult.

- Anticipate and prepare for more complex OSCE stations involving several different tasks.

# 4.6 Thinking ahead: career planning

Phew. It's been a crazy, hectic year with so much to think about. Your brain is probably hurting already from all the things you've seen, heard and learned. If you want to just focus on getting through to finals without worrying about what comes afterwards, then that's totally fair enough and I absolutely don't blame you! If so, feel free to skip this section and enjoy a well-earned drink instead. It's perfectly normal not to have concrete career plans yet – I didn't at this stage – and you shouldn't get stressed out if this is the case. You still have at least two years to decide, as the earliest you can apply for specialty training is during FY2. And plenty of junior doctors defer the decision even further by locuming or taking time out after FY2, so don't let anyone tell you that you need to have your mind made up already!

However, I am also conscious that some students are super-organised and love to plan ahead. Some of you will also have very clear ideas about your future career paths and may be wondering what you can do to boost your prospects of getting into your chosen specialty. If this is the case, then here are the main things you should do to get started:

- Get an overview of all the different medical training options by visiting the websites in **Box 4.11**. Look into 'Person specifications' for the specific details of what each specialty requires.

- Get advice from your medical school, particularly if they offer one-to-one sessions.

- Talk to specialty trainees during your placements and ask for pointers on how to get ahead.

- Get involved in any audits, quality improvement projects, publications or posters which come your way. Audits and QIPs are essential for some specialty applications (although you will have plenty of opportunity to do them in FY1/FY2).

- Enter student prizes and awards at both your medical school and the national level. There are absolutely loads: you've got nothing to lose by going for them, but potentially lots to gain if you win one.

- Attend any conferences, events or further training which are relevant to your chosen specialty.

- For your elective and any 'student-selected' modules or placements, choose something which demonstrates interest in your specialty and which you could discuss in an interview.

- Get involved in student societies for your area of interest.

Finally, don't be disheartened if you're not sure whether you want to go ahead with a career in medicine or even to enter the Foundation Programme. As much as I hope you are feeling inspired to become a doctor, there is absolutely no shame in feeling like you aren't, and you shouldn't try to bottle these feelings up and just hope they go away. Talk it through with your friends and family, get advice from your medical school and ensure you make a careful and considered decision which is right for you. There is also some useful advice on alternative careers from Health Education England[5] and the BMA[6] which you might want to check out. It's **your** future and **your** life: you only get one chance to live it, so do something that makes you feel happy, satisfied and excited to get out of bed in the morning. If that isn't medicine, then find your own path and live it to the full!

**Box 4.11**

### Useful resources for medical career planning

- NHS Health Careers: www.healthcareers.nhs.uk/explore-roles/doctors/roles-doctors
- NHS Specialty Training: https://specialtytraining.hee.nhs.uk/Recruitment
- BMA Careers: https://www.bma.org.uk/advice/career
- The various medical/surgical colleges, such as the Royal College of Physicians: www.rcplondon.ac.uk/education-practice/advice/how-choose-your-medical-specialty
- Or the Royal College of Surgeons: www.rcseng.ac.uk/careers-in-surgery/medical-students/
- Careers articles on the BMJ's students page: www.bmj.com/student

---

5 www.healthcareers.nhs.uk/career-planning/resources/alternative-career-options-medical-students

6 www.bma.org.uk/advice/career/studying-medicine/insiders-guide-to-medical-specialties/alternative-career-choices

# Chapter 5
# Final year

## Contents

# 5.1 What's it all about?

Aaaaaaand... breathe. You made it to the final year of medical school. The hardest years are behind you and the end is finally in sight. Congratulations – it's a huge moment!

I really enjoyed final year but I have to say, it's a bit weird. It feels very different from all the other years because the focus shifts from teaching you loads of new information onto reinforcing and consolidating what you've already been taught in order to get you ready to become an FY1. As well as preparing for finals, there are also multiple other demands on your time, notably Foundation Programme applications, the PSA, the SJT and organising your elective, all of which you will need to juggle alongside your placements and studies. And you may be sent far and wide for your placements, which can feel rather lonely if you're not with your friends. This requires you to be highly independent with your studies, and it can all feel very far removed from the early years of medical school.

There is a lot of variety between medical schools in how final year is structured so I won't dwell on this: you'll find out soon enough how yours is laid out and what's expected of you. You'll need to be very proactive and organised as there are lots of different dates and deadlines which you can't afford to miss, particularly when it comes to Foundation Programme applications and the national exams. You should also make sure you plan your elective in plenty of time, as this is a sweet opportunity to do something amazing before real life kicks in.

Box 5.1

**The key elements of final year**

1. Medical and surgical 'apprenticeships', with an emphasis on shadowing the FY1s
2. ± any new placements: e.g. A&E, anaesthetics, GP
3. Finals
4. Foundation Programme applications
5. SJT
6. PSA
7. Elective

The other major difference between final year and earlier years is that your academic scores no longer count towards your Foundation Programme applications, as we discussed earlier. Essentially, you just need to *pass* all your med school exams, and anything extra is icing on the cake. This fact evokes different reactions in different people: some see it as a great opportunity to finish on a high by acing finals and picking up as

TOP TIP

Be extra organised and proactive in final year. There is lots of paperwork, and dates and deadlines which you really don't want to miss.

many prizes as possible; others want to take their foot off the gas and try to recoup a bit of energy before beginning the grind of a demanding job. For me, having already worked hard and picked up good marks, final year was very liberating as I felt I could relax and enjoy medicine without the added pressure of needing to maximise my EPM. There's also comfort in the fact that you know the drill by this stage: you've got your study techniques locked down, you know how to cope on placements and you've already passed a whole bunch of written exams and OSCEs. Perhaps for the first time, these things have begun to feel familiar instead of mysterious and scary.

I would just add a note of caution: enjoy these feelings but don't let them trip you up so close to the finish line. Plenty of people have to retake final year, which is an experience you'll desperately want to avoid. This is probably the most important message for your last year of medical school:

**Whatever your attitude towards it, just make sure you keep your eye on the ball and find the right balance between enjoying yourself and taking those final steps to develop into a doctor. It's your last chance to convince your medical school that you are up to the standards required for the job – don't give them any opportunity to think otherwise!**

# 5.2 Resources and techniques

We've already covered all the tricks and tactics I deployed to survive medical school, so now it's just a case of using them sensibly in final year. If you're anything like me, you'll be heavily reliant on question banks, flashcards and small, quick-reference books by this point in your studies. Gone are the days of burying your head in long chapters, spending hours on YouTube, making elaborate anatomical drawings and producing reams of your own notes. You've already learned the major building blocks such as anatomy and physiology, and should only be dipping back into these subjects as revision and to clarify things you get wrong or don't understand.

**In general, your focus should now be clinical: what's wrong with this patient and how do I investigate and manage them?**

For this reason, question banks are extremely appealing at this stage and are probably the number one resource used by final-year students. They allow you to relentlessly test yourself to ensure you can spot key symptoms and signs and convert them into a correct diagnosis and management plan. A lot of this is pattern recognition, which you can successfully develop through large volumes of practice exam questions reinforced by flashcards and group study sessions.

But don't forget that finals include OSCEs as well as written exams, so to look the part you will need to keep polishing your pattern recognition on *real patients*, not just on MCQs (also, real patients are a lot more interesting and fun!). There is a tendency among some final-year students to forget this and retreat into a world of doing PassMedicine in your pyjamas. Resist this temptation: get dressed, go into placement and keep clerking and examining as many patients as possible.

A&E, GP and acute medical placements are absolutely ideal for this, as you can get exposure to a huge array of different conditions, preferably without knowing the diagnosis in advance (**Section 5.3.6**). You're doing this for your own benefit now, so don't worry about covering every single bit of the history or examination – try instead to imitate the junior doctors by asking concise questions, doing focused examinations and coming up with succinct differentials and a management plan. Really push yourself to get faster and more efficient at this process, whilst ensuring that you didn't overlook anything important. This won't be easy – it's one of the greatest challenges in all of medicine – but you've got to try!

# 5.3  Clinical placements

## 5.3.1  Medical and surgical assistantships

You will almost certainly have medical and surgical placements in final year but they usually take on a different flavour from previous placements. Now, the emphasis switches from learning new material onto shadowing the FY1s in order to learn what their job is all about. These blocks tend to have names such as 'Assistantships' or 'Preparation for Practice'. It's a response by medical schools to feedback that students felt they hadn't been properly prepared for life as an FY1, and that the step up from final year was too steep. So this type of placement has been brought in to bridge that gap, which seems very sensible to me.

Nevertheless, despite being a good idea in theory, these placements do have some inherent issues which can cause attendances to drop. Here are some of the problems with them:

- Shadowing FY1s can be boring
- You're basically doing their job without getting paid for it!
- They won't necessarily help you pass finals
- If you've already passed finals, then there is no real incentive to show up any more!
- Feeling a bit in no-man's-land: you're not an FY1 yet, but not quite a student any more either.

These points are all reasonable, but I would still encourage you to give these placements a decent go because they will greatly increase your confidence and readiness to start as an FY1 when the time comes around, even if that still feels a little way off. So I will try to help you understand these placements, starting by asking ourselves: just what do FY1s do all day?

## 5.3.2  The life and times of an FY1

I'm sure you've spent plenty of time with FY1s already, but you haven't necessarily imagined yourself in their shoes yet or considered what their whole job entails. So here, in a nutshell, is what FY1s do on a typical day in their job – and what **you** will likely be doing next year:

### Ward days

1. **Mornings:** ward rounds. The FY1 usually documents while a consultant, registrar or SHO sees the patients and devises a plan for their care. This might be on paper or using a COW (computer on wheels), depending on the hospital. The FY1 needs to review and record the latest observations, results and examination findings, note down what was said by the doctor and patient and ensure every part of the plan gets documented. Less commonly, in my hospital at least, the FY1s will see patients by themselves without a senior.

2. **Afternoons:** doing 'jobs'. This means carrying out the plans made during the ward round for each patient. Some can be done during the

round, particularly with electronic systems where it just takes a few clicks to make referrals or order tests, but there will usually be plenty left over at the end. These will often be written out on one page as a 'jobs list', with a little box next to each job so it can be ticked off once it's done (see **Figure 3.4** for a reminder). FY1 ward jobs include, but are not limited to:

**a.** Referring to other specialties for advice or a review of a patient, while doing your best to avoid mentioning that you're an FY1 so that they might actually take you seriously ("Hi I'm **one of the doctors** on the respiratory ward…")

**b.** Doing blood tests, ABGs, cannulas or any other procedures required, or trying to palm these off onto medical students ("Now, I know three FY1s, two SHOs, a registrar and a consultant interventional radiologist using ultrasound guidance all failed at inserting that cannula, but you should **definitely** give it a try…")

**c.** Ordering scans and investigations, and 'chasing' them to make sure they actually happen ("Hi, is that radiology? I've got a patient here who's been waiting for a chest X-ray since 1997. Can I send them down this afternoon please?" "Sure we've got a free slot at … oh wait did you say you're an FY1? Nah fully booked till 2034, sorry pal.")

**d.** Writing discharge summaries and 'TTAs' for patients who are going home. A discharge summary is a description of the main events that took place during a patient's admission, including their diagnosis, management, any changes to their usual medications and the plan for follow-up after discharge. TTA stands for To Take Away (aka TTO / To Take Out), which refers to the medications dispensed for patients to take home with them when they leave.

**e.** Buying coffee and chocolate to ease the pain of writing nine discharge summaries in a row.

**f.** Speaking to pharmacy who have 17 questions about the TTA you just submitted (**Figure 5.1**).

**g.** Discussions with patients and their families. These can be informal conversations in person or over the phone, or more formal family meetings with a senior present. FY1s gather useful collateral information, provide updates, answer questions and sometimes just translate into plain English whatever was said on the ward round ("How much did you understand of what the consultant said to you earlier?" "The bit where he said his name and then the bit where he left." "Riiiiiight then, let's start at the beginning ...")

**h.** Prescribing-related tasks such as reviewing drug charts, clarifying doses and ensuring patients receive VTE prophylaxis (Or, more likely, start looking something up in the **BNF**, get distracted by the FY1 WhatsApp group, totally forget to prescribe the thing then wake up in a cold sweat at 2 a.m. when the realisation hits).

**i.** Fill in annoying automated alerts that pop up in electronic patient record systems, which everyone else has just been overriding because they know some poor sucker like you will fill it in later. (You show them who's boss by ... filling it in later).

**j.** Looking through results of blood tests taken earlier in the day and ordering more for the next morning's phlebotomy round ("Reckon the phlebs will bleed the guy in side room 5 who stabbed that nurse in the eye with a fork?" "Just put him on the list – what's the worst that could happen?").

## On-call days

These involve carrying a bleep and being away from regular ward and day-to-day activities. An FY1 could be:

**1.** Clerking new admissions under the medical or surgical team 'on take', i.e. seeing new patients who came in through A&E or were referred by GPs.

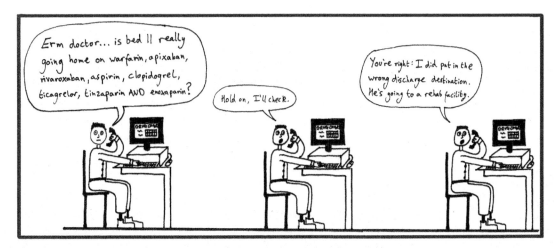

**Figure 5.1: Discharge summaries and 'TTAs' make up a large part of FY1s' workload.** They are usually accompanied by a phone call from pharmacy, who bail you out by picking up your errors.

2. Reviewing new admissions with a consultant, in a process known as 'post take'. This is basically a ward round spread across different locations, but predominantly A&E, in which all new patients are reviewed by a consultant within 24 hours of admission.

3. Carrying out any jobs required for these new admissions, or 'handing them over to' (aka palming them off onto) the ward teams.

4. Doing 'ward cover'. This means being part of a team covering all the medical or surgical wards at night and over the weekends. This involves completing pre-specified tasks handed over by the usual day teams for those wards, as well as any new tasks that arise, such as when nurses bleep to ask you to amend a prescription or come and review a patient who has taken a turn for the worse.

## Clinic days

In some specialties, such as community psychiatry, FY1s are expected to see patients by themselves in clinic. They are usually given plenty of time with each patient and have senior support to discuss concerns and review their management plans. This is not that common, however – wards and on-calls really are the bread and butter of being an FY1 – and it's unlikely you'd be given an assistantship shadowing in this situation. So we don't need to concern ourselves with this for now, but it's something to be aware of when ranking your job preferences.

## 5.3.3  The mindset and skill set of an FY1

It is a sad but little-acknowledged truth that being an FY1 on the ward involves a significant change in mindset (**Figure 5.2**). As a student, you can take a keen interest in patients' stories, diseases, diagnoses and all the other interesting stuff that made you want to do medicine in the first place. As an FY1, on the other hand, you don't have time to indulge in such intellectual luxuries: instead, you become primarily focused on **what needs to be done** for the patients, so that you can get all your work finished, have a lunch break and go home at a reasonable time. Everything else, no matter how interesting, has the potential to be a distraction from your workload. This probably sounds bleak but it's true! That's not to say FY1s don't enjoy themselves or learn and grow as well, but in my experience these aspects are definitely secondary to the day-to-day practicality of just getting stuff done. People will **expect** you to have all the scans chased and bloods ordered; they won't have the same expectations for your intellectual development or enjoyment.

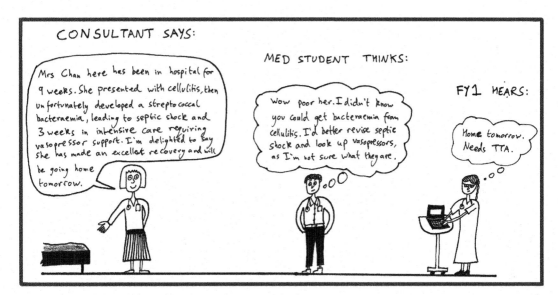

**Figure 5.2: Thinking like an FY1.** Part of the transition from student to junior doctor is to become focused on what needs to be done for the patient here and now, rather than what's happened before.

Of course this isn't your direct concern just **yet**, but it's worth being aware of during your assistantships as it's essential to understanding FY1s, which is the aim of these placements. If there's a really interesting patient with a great history and signs, you can go spend half an hour with them but the FY1 is unlikely to join you because they simply can't spare that amount of time. Likewise observing an interesting procedure such as an ascitic drain insertion: unless they are in the process of learning how to do

**Key skills for FY1s**  **Box 5.2**

- Ability to prioritise tasks
- Being organised and efficient
- Good time management
- Procedures such as bloods, cannulation and ABGs
- Knowledge of commonly prescribed drugs
- Knowing how to navigate your hospital's ecosystem: how and where things happen, and who to speak to to get them done
- Typing quickly without mistakes (if notes are electronic)
- Writing quickly and clearly (if notes are paper)
- Coping with the stress of bleeps and crash calls
- Communicating with patients, families, other specialties and departments
- Summarising information
- Making accurate records of events you have witnessed
- Wheeling COWs through tight spaces without injuring anyone.

**KEY POINT**

> An FY1's main focus is on making sure that everything gets done for the patients. If they enjoy themselves and learn stuff in the process then that's a bonus, but it's sadly not essential for the job!

it themselves, they aren't going to get much out of just watching someone else do it and will be anxious about wasting that time.

Similarly, it's worth considering the knowledge and skills required to be an FY1. So much of the stuff you learned in medical school – anatomy, pathology, physiology and diagnostic reasoning, for example – plays very little role in the day-to-day life of the most junior doctors on a ward (remember that senior doctors usually make the diagnoses and plans; we just implement them). See **Box 5.2** for a realistic list of the skills you will require the most once you start working. I hope this doesn't put you off – FY1 is an important rite of passage and personally I've enjoyed it hugely – but you do need to be aware that there is a lot of admin and boring stuff to do when you are on the wards!

### 5.3.4  How to shadow an FY1

Now you know what an FY1's job entails, we can think about how to go about shadowing them. **Box 5.3** has some top tips.

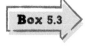

**Box 5.3**

> **Top tips for getting the most out of shadowing an FY1**
>
> - Remember we're humans trying to do a job – be friendly, polite and helpful. Don't get in the way, be annoying or increase our workload!
> - Offer to write in the notes as much as possible instead of just watching us do it, which is boring. Always sign clearly and state your role.
> - Make a few referrals, with help.
> - Do *loads* of procedures.
> - Clerk and examine plenty of patients during on-call shifts.
> - Do a handful of discharge summaries and TTAs just to get the idea but seriously, they are boring so don't do loads.
> - Make yourself part of the team by attending for several days in a row and getting to know the patients, doctors and daily routines. Showing up for the odd day or an hour here and there doesn't make much of an assistantship.
> - Do a mixture of ward days and on-call days (you will probably find the latter much more enjoyable).
> - Join for the odd night shift and/or ward cover: not necessarily the whole thing, but enough to get a feel for it, as the experience can be very different to day shifts.

### 5.3.5 Develop a general examination

As a final-year student, you should now be moving past the stage of spending hours examining each body system in excruciating detail, looking for every clinical sign under the sun. To become less like a student and more like a real doctor, I would suggest you develop a quick general examination on your placements in which you briefly examine all the major body systems in no more than ten minutes (**Figure 5.3**). This is a far more realistic approximation of what real doctors do when they are clerking real patients! Then you can return to examine a system in more detail only if you suspect there is pathology which you need to investigate further. This is something you don't really get taught at medical school but will gradually figure out for yourself in FY1, so hopefully I can speed up that process for you!

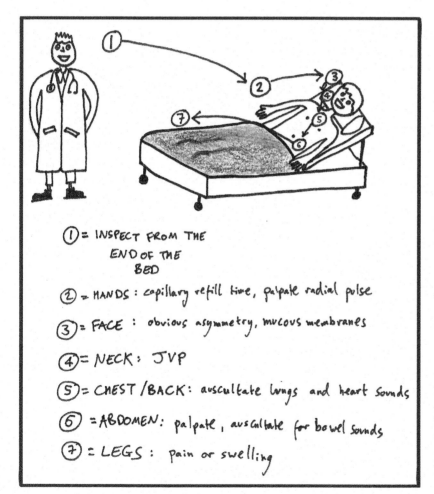

① = INSPECT FROM THE END OF THE BED

② = HANDS : capillary refill time, palpate radial pulse

③ = FACE : obvious asymmetry, mucous membranes

④ = NECK : JVP

⑤ = CHEST / BACK: auscultate lungs and heart sounds

⑥ = ABDOMEN: palpate, auscultate for bowel sounds

⑦ = LEGS : pain or swelling

Figure 5.3: A suggested general examination structure to use when clerking patients on final-year placements. This is *a lot* quicker and more realistic than doing the entire cardiovascular, respiratory, abdominal and neurological examinations you were taught at the start of medical school, with all the fiddly little steps they entail. You should only do the extra steps when you feel they are relevant, not as a routine.

### 5.3.6 New placements: A&E, anaesthetics and GP

As well as assistantships, you may still have a few new placements to contend with in final year which you've either not experienced before, or experienced in a much less hands-on way. This will depend on your medical school, but in my case these comprised A&E and anaesthetics, both for the first time, and GP which I had previously experienced as an observer but in which I was now expected to see patients on my own.

A&E is basically the perfect placement for final year as it allows you to see loads of patients and practise a wide range of skills whilst having a timetable that is usually quite flexible and can be tailored to your needs. Show up at a time that suits you, find out how to access the list of patients who are waiting to be seen, then ask confidently whether you can see one of them first and present it to a junior before they see the patient themselves. Get feedback on your presentation, then go with the doctor and observe how they do it: what was the same as how you did it? What was different? What did you do well and what could you have done better? This is an *amazing* learning exercise and absolutely fantastic preparation for finals OSCEs.

You don't need to stay for ages: A&E is so busy with people coming and going that no one will really notice whether you're there or not. If you stayed for just three hours, you could see three patients in this time and do a really thorough job on each one, including looking through all their blood tests and imaging and talking it through with the junior doctor. Do this a few times per week and you could be up to 10 or 15 patients who you saw by yourself – potentially as many as 50 by the end of your placement. Believe me, this will make an absolutely **huge** difference to your performance in finals and you will learn loads and feel a lot more satisfied in the process!

Anaesthetics is another fantastic placement for final year, if you've not already had it. Despite working in a life-or-death specialty riddled with brown-trouser moments, anaesthetists are a remarkably chilled-out

**TOP TIP**

Anaesthetics placements provide some of the best teaching in all of medical school and are a golden opportunity to practise your procedural skills under supervision. Make the most of them!

> A&E and GP placements provide a fantastic opportunity to see a large volume of patients by yourself, perhaps for the first time. Use this to build up your confidence, pattern recognition and diagnostic reasoning in preparation for finals OSCEs and on-call shifts as an FY1.

TOP TIP

bunch. They love to teach students and are extremely generous with their time: if you're sitting with them during an operation, they'll potentially chat to you for the entire two or three hours while the patient is on the table and will often let you choose which topics you want to discuss. I guarantee there is no other specialty where registrars and consultants will give you this much face time in a clinical setting (most surgeons will barely give you the time of day), so I really urge you to make the most of it! As well as covering specific anaesthetics topics, you can also grab the opportunity to discuss virtually any element of physiology or pharmacology, which is great revision for finals. Hanging out with anaesthetists also offers some much-needed practice at procedures such as cannulation, so you can boost your skills and confidence ahead of becoming an FY1.

Like me, you probably already did a GP placement earlier in medical school, but the big difference in final year is that you should be allowed to start seeing patients by yourself. This is daunting at first but it's brilliant for developing your clinical and communication skills and diagnostic reasoning. If your supervisors aren't keen on letting you see patients by yourself, I'd really encourage you to push for it because it's infinitely more informative than just sitting in the corner observing the GP, which is starting to get a little boring by this stage of your training! Show them that you are professional, polite and competent and can handle this responsibility. You're not expected to know everything or to be super-quick, but you are expected to show up on time, look the part and be respectful to patients. Don't worry too much about 'getting things wrong', as you will usually have an opportunity to discuss each case with a supervisor after you've finished seeing them. Concentrate more on doing a focused history and examination and coming up with differentials and a management plan ready to present to your supervisor. Like with A&E, this is absolutely invaluable experience and will stand you in great stead whatever career path you choose later on.

### 5.3.7 Summary

In this section, we have looked at what to expect from clinical placements in your final year. The key points are:

- You will probably have to 'shadow' an FY1 on medicine and/or surgery: these placements aren't perfect but they do have a lot of positives and will make you feel better prepared to begin work as a junior doctor.
- Put some effort into understanding the roles, responsibilities, mindset and skill set of FY1s.
- Try to help them out rather than getting in their way.
- Make sure you experience on-call shifts as well as daily ward work.
- Develop a quick general examination to use when clerking patients, which is more realistic of how real doctors do it.
- A&E, anaesthetics and GP placements can be brilliant for your learning and building up your confidence and pattern recognition with real patients.
- Try to see patients by yourself as much as possible: this will help a lot with finals OSCEs.

# 5.4  The Foundation Programme

Hands up who enjoys filling in paperwork, compiling spreadsheets, reading long and tedious PDFs and battling with clunky websites with a poor user interface? That's exactly why you went into medicine, right? For the love of admin and outmoded tech?

If you raised your hand to the above, then you are going to **love** applying to the Foundation Programme. Everyone else is going to want to gouge their eyes out with a blunt pencil, put their eyes back in, then gouge them out again. Forewarned is forearmed.

Yes, Foundation Programme applications are by far and away one of the **least** enjoyable elements of final year and probably all of medical school. However, they are entirely unavoidable should you wish to practise medicine in the UK, so I'm afraid you will just have to deal with them! Let's take just a **brief** look at how it all works – any more than that and I might start reaching for the pencil myself.

Be extremely organised and proactive when it comes to Foundation Programme applications. No matter how unenjoyable you find the process, you will need to engage with it and pore over the websites and information with a fine-toothed comb to ensure you don't miss anything.

TOP TIP

## 5.4.1 Overview

The UK Foundation Programme is the national employment and training scheme for junior doctors fresh out of medical school. Everyone gets assigned to a two-year programme, known as Foundation Year 1 (FY1 or F1) and Foundation Year 2 (FY2 or F2), which is "intended to equip doctors with the generic skills and professional capabilities to progress to specialty training".[1]

The first things to decide are whether you want to apply at all and if so, whether to the main Foundation Programme or the Academic Foundation Programme. The latter is suited to people considering a career in research or academia.[2] There are important differences in the timelines and processes, so make sure you research the academic option thoroughly if you are considering it.

**Timeline for applying to the UK Foundation Programme**

Box 5.4

This is intended as a general guide: please check the website for specific dates for your year.
- June–September: register and submit documentation
- September: all jobs become available to view online. EPM scores released by medical schools, grouped by decile
- December–January: sit the SJT
- February: deadline for ranking your deanery choices
- Early March: SJT scores released. Applicants assigned to deaneries based on overall Application Scores
- Late March: deadline for ranking jobs within your deanery
- April: job matches released
- May–August: pre-employment checks and paperwork with your employer
- June: provisional registration with GMC
- Late July: shadowing/induction period
- First Wednesday of August (aka Black Wednesday)[3]: begin work.

---

1  www.foundationprogramme.nhs.uk/content/2-year-foundation-programme
2  www.foundationprogramme.nhs.uk/content/academic-training
3  It's known as Black Wednesday because researchers have shown a small but statistically significant increase in death rates during the first week that the new foundation doctors begin work. The tabloids love crowing about this fact: expect to see a bunch of articles warning people not to attend hospital that week. But fewer attendances will mean less work for you, so let's not complain about it, eh?

For our purposes, we'll stick with the main programme as it's by far the larger group. In this, your two years are made up of four-monthly rotations, so you will do three jobs in FY1 and three jobs in FY2, for a total of six jobs. Usually, all six jobs will be assigned up front, so the whole two years are mapped out for you before you start (unless you make swaps, which is often possible).

Around 8000 medical graduates get placed into the Foundation Programme each year, according to their website. It's a competitive process, with jobs assigned on the basis of your 'Application Score'; see **Figure 5.4** for a reminder of how this is calculated. Essentially, you rank jobs in the order that you want them, then the person with the highest score is given their first choice, then the person with the second-highest score gets their first choice if it's still available or their second choice if not, and so on. The higher your score, the more likely you are to get one of your top choices. The lower your score, the further down your list of preferences you are likely to end up.

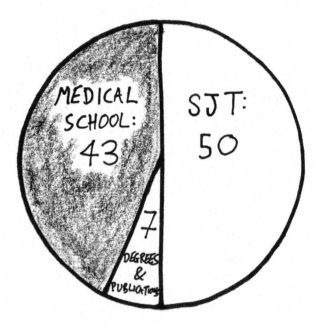

**Figure 5.4: Scoring system for entry to the UK Foundation Programme.**
Your medical school performance is worth 43 out of 100 points, then your 'educational achievements' (publications and other degrees) are worth another 7 points. Together these are known as the Educational Performance Measure (EPM), worth 50 points in total. The remaining 50 points come from the Situational Judgement Test (SJT), a one-off exam focusing on professionalism, ethics and law.

## 5.4.2 The application process

From your perspective, the job application process is essentially split into two parts. The first decision is **where** you want to work once you graduate. For this, the UK is divided into deaneries (they're actually now called Units of Application, or UoAs, but this is a piece of jargon too far for me), which comprise groups of hospitals, clinics and general practices within a defined geographical area. Deaneries are extremely variable in size: for example, London is divided into three separate deaneries, whereas **all of Scotland** is a single deanery. So are Wales and Northern Ireland. Your choice of deanery will probably come quite naturally, but see **Box 5.5** for a few factors to consider. There is also a lot of information available to help you through the Foundation Programme website, the individual deanery and Foundation school websites, and from your medical school.

Once you've been assigned a deanery, the much more complex and fiddly part is ranking all the different jobs within it. There are usually hundreds: in my case, last year, I had some 340 different options to choose from. This is where you will need to get deep into spreadsheets: many students end up constructing very elaborate lists with complex colour coding and clever macros to help them make sense of it all. Many of the considerations from **Box 5.5** will still apply at this point; see **Box 5.6** for some more specific pointers on how to choose your jobs. You should also draw on your experiences from medical school, particularly if you are remaining in the same location where you attended placements.

**What factors should I consider when choosing my deanery?**   **Box 5.5**

- Proximity to home, friends and family, or any other personal factors.
- Opportunity to live and work somewhere new: either just for a couple of years, or with a view to settling longer-term.
- Costs of living, commuting and other expenses (your salary will be roughly the same wherever, but it'll stretch much further outside London, for example).
- Competitiveness of that deanery: how likely am I to get into it, based on my scores?
- Competitiveness of jobs: how likely am I to get the one I want within the deanery?
- If my scores aren't great and I have to be pragmatic: would I rather get a great location but crappy jobs, or vice versa?
- Specific jobs: does this deanery usually have lots of jobs in the specialties I want to work in longer-term?
- Specific locations: is there a particular hospital or department I want to work in for the advancement of my career?
- Training and education: does that deanery have a reputation for supporting, training and looking after its juniors?
- Pace of work: am I better suited to big inner-city hospitals or smaller district generals?
- Consider *all* the options properly: you need to rank every deanery in order of preference, so don't just optimistically rank your top five then pick the rest at random or you may get a nasty surprise if the SJT doesn't go as well as you'd hoped...
- Special circumstances: having children or significant caring responsibilities ensures your deanery of choice, but you'll still have to compete normally for the jobs within it. So, depending how large the deanery is, you can still end up a long way from home.

Box 5.6

**What factors should I consider when ranking my jobs?**

1. **The hospitals:** are they nice places to work? Busy? Large? Easy to get to? Supportive? What sort of population do they serve?
2. **The departments:** are they nice places to work? Well staffed? Do they have particular expertise or interests? Good reputation for teaching, training and developing juniors?
3. **The specialties/jobs:** which are you interested in doing in the long term? Which do you want to experience just for four months? Which do you never want to do? Which are best suited to your skills and personality?
4. **The order:** do I want to ease into FY1 or go straight into the deep end? Are there particular placements I want to do *before* applying to specialty training? (applications are made towards the beginning of FY2, so you will have two remaining placements which you won't have experienced when you apply).
5. **The rotas:** what are the hours? What's the salary? Will you have to work nights and weekends? If so, how many? What's the spread of on-calls versus ward work versus clinics?
6. **Potential for swaps:** don't be too downhearted if you don't get the jobs you wanted as there is often potential to swap with other FY1s. Each deanery has its own rules on this: try to find out in advance, so you have this option up your sleeve if the job allocations don't go as you'd hoped.

By this stage you will have received your SJT score, so you know your Application Score in its entirety. This gives you a better idea of how highly you are placed within your deanery, and therefore which of your preferences you are realistically likely to get. This determines roughly how many jobs you need to rank: if you're the top-scoring applicant in your deanery, for example, you will get your first choice so there is no point agonising over the other 339 options. If you're towards the bottom, you will need to rank all 340 options to cover all your bases.

## 5.4.3 Do your research

An absolutely essential step in applying for the Foundation Programme is to properly research your choices of hospital and jobs. Don't just assume that the FY1 geriatrics job in hospital A is the same as the FY1 geriatrics job in hospital B, for example. They might be completely different working environments, with differing hours, levels of staffing, stress and support. Leave this to chance, and you might end up with a nasty surprise on day one.

The best thing you can do is speak to the current crop of FY1s at the hospitals you are considering applying to. They are usually delighted to help and will tell you **exactly** what the pros and cons of that hospital are, including which departments to rank highly and which to avoid at all costs. Trust me, this information exists, it just isn't written down anywhere so you need to talk to people to find it! Reach out to contacts through social media, friends of friends, medical school networks, whatever you can do to track down someone who might chat to you over a coffee or on the phone. There is usually a Facebook group for the deanery in which people ask about swaps and accommodation, so you might be able to find someone that way. If that doesn't work, you can try contacting the hospital's education department or Foundation Programme directors to see if they'll put you in touch with some current FY1s. And if all else fails, just ring up the hospital and ask to be put through to one of the FY1s on call. They might not react amazingly at first, especially if they are extremely busy, but be super-apologetic about it, explain that you've exhausted all your other options and ask if you can grab their email address so they can respond at a more suitable time. The worst-case scenario is a complete stranger gets annoyed and hangs up on you – this is **vastly** better than risking committing a year of your life to a hospital that makes you miserable!

Another option I'd highly recommend is to attend any events put on by your deanery or foundation school. They usually run a fair where all the different hospitals have stalls with information, which can help you learn more about your options. They often bring along a few of the current FY1s to chat to you: this is great if you've not previously managed to track one down, but do be aware that you may not get the most honest appraisal if they are manning an official stall and standing next to someone senior when you speak to them!

A final note of caution: even with the best research possible, things might deviate from what you expect. At my current hospital, the policy when I was applying was that FY1s didn't work nights: this sounded like a win to me, and was definitely a factor in my ranking it at the top. I showed up on day one and – whaddya know – the policy had changed and we were the first batch of FY1s to work nights at Barnet Hospital! I was pretty annoyed about it at first, but I can honestly say that my night shifts have been fantastic and I have learned a huge amount from them. Although the schedule is obviously disruptive to daily life, I've found the shifts themselves to be generally quieter and far less pressurised, with more support, teaching and a stronger sense of camaraderie between the team. So keep an open mind – you just never know how things are going to turn out!

# 5.5 Situational Judgement Test (SJT)

## 5.5.1 What's it all about?

The Situational Judgement Test is a national exam you have to take in final year as part of your Foundation Programme application. It's all about professionalism, ethics and law, testing how you would behave in certain situations in the workplace. It's unlike any other exam you take at medical school and the stakes are high because of the impact it will have on the next two years of your life and career, so it's vital to engage properly with it. As we saw in Section 5.4.1, the SJT accounts for a whopping 50 of 100 marks on your Foundation Programme application score: that's more than your entire performance throughout medical school, which is worth just 43.

**KEY POINT**

> The SJT is worth up to 50 marks out of 100 on your Foundation Programme application. The average SJT score is around 40.

The SJT is relatively new: it was introduced in 2012–13 along with the Educational Performance Measure as part of a drive to standardise the process of ranking students for the Foundation Programme and minimise variation between medical schools. Previously there was an application form with short essay-type questions which you had to fill in in your own time. This form was felt by the Department of Health to be an unreliable method of ranking students and potentially open to plagiarism, while students apparently found the whole process unfair and stressful.[4,5] So the powers that be scrapped it and brought in the SJT instead. So now everyone's happy, right?

Well, no. Far from it. They're about as happy as I was last night when my two-year-old son did a poo in the bath which I had to fish out. Very not happy indeed. We'll look shortly at why the SJT evokes such strong feelings. But first we need to understand exactly what it entails and how best to go about preparing for it.

---

4 www.medschools.ac.uk/our-work/assessment/situational-judgement-test
5 https://isfp.org.uk/isfp-timeline/

## 5.5.2 **What does it look like?**

The SJT is a one-off exam lasting 2 hours and 20 minutes and comprising 70 questions (ten of those questions are fake 'pilot questions' which don't count towards your score, but you don't know which questions are real and which are fake so this information is of no practical value whatsoever). It's all done on good old-fashioned paper – who needs trees anyway? – with those boxy answer sheets that get read by a malevolent robot who instantly fails you for not using an HB pencil. It's supposed to test you across nine domains which have been deemed to be important for life as an FY1:

1. Commitment to professionalism

2. Coping with pressure

3. Effective communication

4. Learning and professional development

5. Organisation and planning

6. Patient focus

7. Problem-solving and decision-making

8. Self-awareness and insight

9. Working effectively as part of a team.

There are two sections in the SJT:

1. Ranking questions: you are given a scenario and five possible options for how you should respond. You need to rank these options from 'most appropriate' to 'least appropriate'. The marking system for these questions is a bit complex, but essentially they give you partial credit for getting things nearly-but-not-quite right. You will score between 8 and 20 for each question, provided you fill it in correctly. There are 46 of these questions – around two-thirds of the exam.

2. MCQs: you are given a scenario and have to pick three out of eight possible answers. You get 4 marks for each correct one you pick and a big fat zero for incorrect ones, so you can potentially score 0, 4, 8 or 12 for each question. There are 24 of these questions – around one-third of the exam.

**Box 5.7**

**Example SJT ranking question[6]**

You are just finishing a busy shift on the Acute Admissions Unit. Your FY1 colleague who is due to replace you for the evening shift leaves a message with the nurse in charge that she will be 15 to 30 minutes late. There is only a 30-minute overlap between your timetables to hand over to your colleague. You need to leave on time as you have a social engagement to attend with your partner.

**Rank in order** the following actions in response to this situation (1 = most appropriate; 5 = least appropriate)

A. Make a list of the patients under your care on the AAU, detailing their outstanding issues, leaving this in the doctors' office when your shift ends and then leave at the end of your shift.

B. Quickly go around each of the patients on the AAU, leaving an entry in the notes highlighting the major outstanding issues relating to each patient and then leave at the end of your shift.

C. Make a list of patients and outstanding investigations to give to your colleague as soon as she arrives.

D. Ask your specialty trainee if you can leave a list of your patients and their outstanding issues with him to give to your colleague when she arrives and then leave at the end of your shift.

E. Leave a message for your partner explaining that you will be 30 minutes late.

**Box 5.8**

**Example SJT multiple choice question[6]**

You review a patient on the surgical ward who has had an appendicectomy done earlier in the day. You write a prescription for strong painkillers. The staff nurse challenges your decision and refuses to give the medication to the patient.

Choose the **THREE most appropriate** actions to take in this situation:

A. Instruct the nurse to give the medication to the patient

B. Discuss with the nurse why she disagrees with the prescription

C. Ask a senior colleague for advice

D. Complete a clinical incident form

E. Cancel the prescription on the nurse's advice

F. Arrange to speak to the nurse later to discuss your working relationship

G. Write in the medical notes that the nurse has declined to give the medication

H. Review the case again.

6 Examples from: http://sjt.foundationprogramme.nhs.uk/sample

## 5.5.3 How to prepare

There is a pervasive myth which does the rounds at medical school, in which people say you can't prepare for the SJT. They claim it's supposed to test innate attributes which you either have or you don't, and therefore there's no point revising for it. Others say it's not worth preparing for because it's easy: it's testing your common sense and basic human decency, so unless you're the next Harold Shipman you should be fine on the day.

I don't know where these ideas have come from but to be frank they are complete bollocks. For me, the notion that you can't prepare for the SJT ranks right up there with climate change denial and 'vaccines cause autism' among society's most stupid and dangerous ideas. Of course you can prepare for it – indeed you **must** if you want to do as well as possible. Yes, it's different to other exams because you're not learning new **knowledge** per se, but you are learning a new **skill** which needs practice. And you can **definitely**, **100%** train your brain to process the questions quicker, spot recurring patterns and learn certain principles.

The good news is the preparation process doesn't take too long: I probably spent about six weeks on it and found that my practice scores and speed both improved substantially over that time. Here's how I suggest you go about it:

- Start with a brief overview of the exam by reading the websites and intro chapters of the books in **Table 5.1**. Familiarise yourself with the two different sections and exactly how the marking schemes work. It's also worth skimming the GMC guidance to extract the major points about what attributes they think make a good doctor (only read the whole thing if you are suffering from insomnia or have sadomasochistic tendencies).

- Once you've got the gist of it, go straight into doing the official practice papers under timed conditions. Note down your marks and how long you took.

- Next, spend a serious amount of time going through the explanations and rationales provided, either on your own or with friends. Look very carefully at which questions you bombed on and exactly why you dropped marks. This is the single most valuable exercise you can do as part of your SJT prep so don't skimp on it.

- Extrapolate the overarching **general principles** from these official explanations and write notes for yourself, so that you can apply the principles to any question in future. You will quickly see that even though the scenarios vary, there are common recurring themes such as how to raise safety concerns, how to deal with unprofessional colleagues, how to ensure effective handover, and so on. Develop your own mental framework for dealing with these situations, based on the principles you developed from the official practice papers. One good general principle is to always make the care of the patient your first concern – you won't go far wrong with that – but you'll need to work out others for yourself.

- In ranking questions, there are often one or two blindingly obvious options and then the rest is a grey area where the other options seem equally good or bad as each other. Let's borrow from cricket terminology and call this the corridor of uncertainty (**Figure 5.5**). Really focus on the corridor when developing your general principles as you can pick up a lot of extra marks by ranking these iffy options correctly. So when working through the official answers and rationales, don't just settle for ranking A and C correctly then guessing the rest – also ask yourself: okay B, D and E all seemed like reasonable options to me,

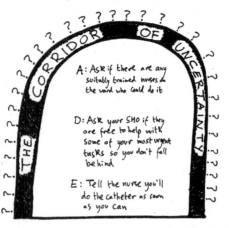

Q: You are the FY1 on call. You are bleeped by a nurse asking you to catheterise a patient on her ward. She says it is urgent but is vague on details. You have a long list of other tasks that need completing, some of which are also urgent. Rank in order the following actions: (1= most appropriate; 5 = least appropriate)

OBVIOUSLY RIGHT

B: Ask the nurse for more information about the patient and look up their electronic record. Once you know the details, prioritise the task in order of clinical urgency. Politely ask the nurse to gather the necessary equipment in the meantime.

CORRIDOR OF UNCERTAINTY

A: Ask if there are any suitably trained nurses on the ward who could do it

D: Ask your SHO if they are free to help with some of your most urgent tasks so you don't fall behind

E: Tell the nurse you'll do the catheter as soon as you can

OBVIOUSLY WRONG

C: Stop what you're doing, gather the equipment then track down the nurse and repeatedly flog her with the catheter to teach her a lesson for bleeping you about such an annoying task. Live stream this to Facebook for bants.

**Figure 5.5: Lots of SJT ranking questions have a couple of obvious answers, then several equally reasonable-sounding options in the middle.** This grey zone, aka the corridor of uncertainty, can cumulatively cost you a lot of marks in the exam if you don't rank them in the right order. So it's well worth putting some serious time and effort into understanding exactly why the examiners thought one option was better than another.

but why **exactly** did they think B was better than E which was better than D? Or, conversely (and this is often the case with SJT questions): I thought B, D and E were all bad options, but why **exactly** was one worse than the others?

- Always remember that they are asking what you **should** do in a particular situation, not what you **would** do. This is a small but absolutely crucial difference. They are effectively asking you to set aside realism, your own instincts and stuff you have seen actual doctors do and instead pretend you are some sort of saintly super-FY1 from another dimension who does absolutely everything by the book. Or, to borrow a popular phrase: what would Jesus do? This is the mindset to adopt when answering SJT questions (**Figure 5.6**).

- Read the questions carefully. This might sound like bog-standard generic advice for any exam, but in the SJT you really do need to look at **exactly** what information is provided, right down to individual words. You cannot extrapolate, fill in gaps or make assumptions: they want you to respond to the scenario precisely as they've presented it. So if the scenario leaves you wanting more information – say you stumble into an argument between colleagues and don't know the background – then proceed cautiously as someone who does not have all the information to hand, rather than rushing into decisive next steps. Conversely, if it overtly states that a colleague is drunk on the job, for example, then you can take that as a fact and prioritise immediate action to protect patient safety rather than waiting to gather more information.

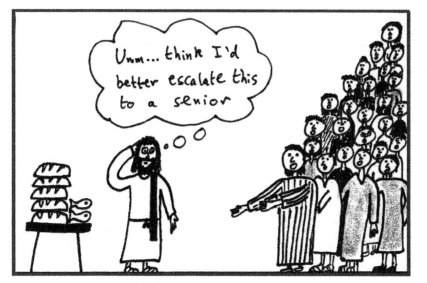

Figure 5.6: When answering SJT questions, ask yourself not "What would a real FY1 do in this situation?" but rather "What would Jesus do in this situation?" That seems to be the level of ethical and professional practice they're aiming at.

- Consider the **order** in which you should do things. Often they will give you five options which all sound like really good things to do, but if you look carefully at the question you'll realise they are asking which you would do **first** or **most urgently**. This is a common pitfall.

- Practise under time pressure. This will be intense on the day so you need to get used to it right from the start. There is no negative marking for getting things wrong, so it's essential to attempt every question even if you guess. Leaving things blank, by contrast, will see you haemorrhage marks faster than blood from a ruptured AAA.

**Table 5.1: SJT resources**

| Official practice papers | Two are available from: http://sjt.foundationprogramme.nhs.uk |
|---|---|
| Official reading material | • *Good Medical Practice* from the GMC: www.gmc-uk.org/ethical-guidance/ethical-guidance-for-doctors/good-medical-practice. This page also has links to interactive scenarios about the content. GMC guidance on consent and confidentiality is also relevant, along with *Tomorrow's Doctors*.<br>• The SJT monograph: https://isfp.org.uk/sjt-monograph/ |
| Unofficial books | • *Oxford Assess and Progress: Situational Judgement Test*<br>• *Get Ahead! The Situational Judgement Test*<br>• *350 Questions for the Situational Judgement Test*<br>• *Pass the Situational Judgement Test: A Guide for Medical Students*<br>• *Situational Judgement Test for the Foundation Years Programme* |
| Unofficial websites and reading material | • Student BMJ: Passing the Situational Judgement Test: www.bmj.com/content/349/sbmj.g6124<br>• http://imperialendo.co.uk/sjt/sjt.htm - has a mock exam as well<br>• Geeky Medics: Top Tips for the Situational Judgement Test (SJT): www.geekymedics.com/top-tips-for-the-situational-judgement-test-sjt/<br>• EMedica: www.emedica.co.uk/bmjsjt.htm<br>• BMJ Learning webinar: www.learning.bmj.com/learning/module-intro/prepare-effectively-situational-judgment-test.html?locale=en_GB&moduleId=10060866 |
| Unofficial online question banks | • PassMedicine<br>• PasTest<br>• OnExamination |

- Once you've gone through the official practice papers in detail, you can use unofficial resources (***Table 5.1***) to practise a large volume of questions, but it's very important that you take the exact answers and rationales with a pinch of salt and do not base your general principles on them. We'll see why in **Section 5.5.4**. **Do not** write your own questions either! And don't go crazy spending loads of money on books and revision courses – it's unnecessary in my opinion and you will never use them again! Use whichever books are in your med school library, plus online material you can get for free or are already subscribed to through question banks.

- Redo all the official practice papers in the days immediately before the exam to ensure your scores and timings have improved since the first time you did them. Use the paper answer sheet and a pencil for your last couple of practice run-throughs (you can download and print it from the SJT website). This will really get you in the zone for the day itself and ensure you can mark the answers quickly and accurately for both sections of the exam.

## 5.5.4 Opinions, opinions, opinions

I went through a very frustrated phase while preparing for the SJT, which I'd like to try and help you to avoid. It occurred around halfway through my preparations, when I felt confident with the content, style and structure of the exam but found my performance on unofficial practice questions had plateaued. I was getting confused by the rationales provided and couldn't understand why I was still dropping marks. I thought a lot about this and eventually had an epiphany which got me back on track. My realisation was this:

> **No matter how much they dress it up in fancy terminology about being objective and evidence-based, the SJT is fundamentally a subjective exercise where the 'correct' answers merely reflect the opinions and beliefs of whoever wrote the question.**

It's an exam about how you should behave in particular workplace situations – well, there are millions of doctors on this earth, and each is a unique human being with their own thoughts and ideas who would behave differently when confronted when a specific series of events. Of course there are general rules we all follow, but when it comes to small details like whether your first port of call should be your registrar, the on-call pharmacist or a fellow FY1 when you are unsure about a prescription, well, the truth is you can make a good case for any of them. Yet this is exactly the sort of scenario that can cost you several marks if you rank them in the 'wrong' order.

This explains why people got really angry during an introductory lecture to the SJT at my medical school. This lecture included a few practice questions the lecturer had written herself, and she explained her rationales. One of these met with disagreement from a student about why D was actually a better option than E, then someone else pitched in to argue why B was in fact better, then someone else put forth the case for A. These were all intelligent people making reasonable arguments – there was a lot of back and forth before it eventually descended into farce. The lecturer got annoyed, gave up and said something to the effect of "Look, that's my answer, now let's just move on". Well, as you can imagine that didn't really satisfy anyone, she lost the crowd and we all left the lecture feeling more confused and stressed than when we went in.

My point, ultimately, is this: you can use all the different books, websites and revision courses you like, but know that the official practice papers, and the GMC guidance on which they are based, are the **only resources you can absolutely trust** because they're written by the same people who will write your questions on the day. Everything else just introduces more opinions from different people, which often contradict each other, muddy the waters and leave you feeling confused and frustrated. This is why you should spend by far the lion's share of your time on the official practice papers and go through their rationales/explanations in great detail when developing your general rules and principles. This is also why you shouldn't write your own practice questions – you will just confuse yourself even more!

I'm not saying you shouldn't use unofficial resources, but do so just to provide a larger quantity of practice questions for you to improve your speed and pattern recognition, not to hone your general principles. Accept that they will give conflicting advice and that you will inevitably drop marks on them, particularly when ranking iffy options in the corridor of uncertainty (see **Figure 5.5**). When this happens, and an unofficial rationale contradicts a principle you had developed from the official papers, just shrug your shoulders, accept it as a difference in opinion and move on. Never go too deep into the rationales provided by unofficial resources or change your overarching principles because of them, because this will only throw you off course. As long as your performance on the **official** papers is improving, then you are heading in the right direction. This is why I was getting so frustrated for a while, and I felt a lot happier once I figured it out!

> You can use unofficial resources to practise answering large volumes of SJT questions but you *cannot* rely on the explanations and rationales they provide, so don't get wound up by them. The official papers are the only source you can really trust when developing your general principles and assessing your performance.

**KEY POINT**

## 5.5.5  SJT strategy

There are two elements of strategy to consider for the SJT on the day. The first is timekeeping: this is the major challenge with the exam as the questions are often long and time-consuming to read. You can also accidentally blow a lot of time weighing up options in the corridor of uncertainty which all seem just as good or bad as each other, so try to avoid falling into this trap. You've got around two minutes per question so keep a close eye on the clock and keep pushing yourself forwards. It's essential to at least attempt every question, as you will drop far more marks for leaving things blank than you will for guessing wrongly.

The second issue is whether to complete the ranking questions or MCQs first. Most people will naturally just do them in the order they come – ranking questions, then MCQs – but see **Box 5.9** for the argument for doing it the other way around. Personally, I bought into this argument and did the MCQs first, but it's really a matter of your own preference. Whichever way you do it, make your decision in plenty of time and practise so you are completely comfortable with it on the day.

## 5.5.6  Controversy about the SJT

We've covered the main points about the SJT itself: what it entails and how to prepare for it. But our discussion would not be complete without also looking at some of the criticisms and tensions that surround this exam and cause a lot of angst for medical students. Here are the main objections to the SJT in its current form:

1. It's inherently subjective (see **Section 5.5.4**). Just because the examiners thought you should finish taking the blood samples before talking to the relatives, or bleep a registrar rather than an SHO, or whatever, that doesn't make it factually correct.

**Box 5.9**

**The rationale for doing part two of the SJT before part one, i.e. the MCQs before the ranking questions**

It's up to you whether or not to do this, but do at least give it some consideration and make a decision in plenty of time.
- **Reminder:** part one gives you five different options to rank in order. There are 46 questions, scoring between 8 and 20 marks each.
  - Based on the large volume of practice questions I did, the most common scores when attempting questions properly are 18, 16 and 14.
  - Even if you blindly guess a question, the way the marking scheme works means the lowest you are likely to score is 12 (you'd be very unlucky to get 8 or 10).
  - In general terms, therefore, you will tend to drop 2–6 points on every question you attempt properly, and the worst-case scenario is you drop 8 by guessing.
- **Reminder:** part two gives you eight different options from which you pick three correct ones. There are 24 questions, scoring 12, 8, 4 or 0 each.
  - The most common scores when attempting questions properly are 12 and 8, as there are usually two fairly obvious answers for 4 marks each.
  - If you blindly guess a question, you can easily score 0 or 4.
  - In general terms, therefore, you will tend to drop 0–4 points on every question you attempt properly, but the worst-case scenario is you drop 12 by guessing.
- **In summary:** questions in part two will cost you more marks by guessing than those in part one. They can also take you longer, as they have more different options to read and consider.
- **Conclusion:** it is therefore worthwhile doing part two *first*, so that you can devote your full attention to the questions when time is less pressured. Or to put it another way: if you are running out of time towards the end of the SJT and have to guess some questions, it's safer to be guessing on part one than part two as you will lose fewer marks.

2. It's far too heavily weighted, with 50 points compared to 43 for the EPM. How on earth can it count for more than the ***entirety*** of medical school?? This is deeply unfair on people who have worked their nuts off for six years yet can jeopardise it all with a poor showing on the SJT. On the flip side, it's a potentially massive 'get out of jail free' card for people who have barely lifted a finger throughout medical school.

**3.** It's a one-off exam which you can't resit without some seriously good extenuating circumstances. This is pretty harsh on those who are unwell, distracted by other life events, or simply having an off day.

**4.** The stakes are too high. Is there any other profession which can force its graduates to live **anywhere in the country for the next two years** based largely on the results of a single exam? Answers on a postcard please.

**5.** You are often being asked to choose between several answers which all seem right, or all seem wrong. This feels a lot like splitting hairs. At the end of the day, if you know something is wrong and you wouldn't do it, does it really matter if it's **more** wrong than something else which you also wouldn't do?

**6.** Questions can feel very artificial. Re-reading the practice papers now that I'm an actual real-life FY1, yes I do recognise lots of the scenarios as being realistic but lots of others feel highly contrived and unrepresentative of real life. Particularly when the **should do** clearly differs from what you know real doctors **would do**, and in fact **do do** on a daily basis.

**7.** It's yet more stress and workload. Some students will spend months preparing for the SJT: couldn't this be better spent working towards finals or on the wards learning, you know, the actual business of how doctors go about their jobs and apply their judgement to real-life situations?

**8.** What's it really testing? The implication is that the SJT is somehow the yin to the yang of academic performance – that it tests whether or not you are a 'good doctor' as well as knowing the sciencey stuff. But last I checked, there is no objective consensus as to what makes a good doctor and there certainly isn't any proof that it correlates with SJT scores. Surely observing students in OSCEs and their real-life interactions with patients on placements is a better judge of character?

I guess I've revealed my true feelings towards the SJT with the list above. In truth I've actually toned it down: I had to scoff an entire crate of lorazepam to write that without wanting to rip the head off the nearest kitten. And I was lying about my son's poo in the bath: that did not make me **anywhere near** as pissed off as the SJT did. I'd gladly fish a turd out of the bath every day for the rest of my life if it spared future generations of medical students from having half their Foundation Programme scores based on this exam.

But those are my own issues, for which I shall endeavour to seek therapy. I'm just telling you so you know you're not alone if you resent it and think it's unfair. In fact these feelings seem to be common: in a survey of 51 final-year students, there were generally low levels of agreement with the statement that the SJT is a worthwhile method of assessing our professional attributes (across five of the domains it is supposed to test, average scores ranged from 2.29 to 2.61 on a scale where 1 = strongly disagree and 5 = strongly agree). The survey respondents also provided some choice comments, for which I can only commend them.[7]

**"I cannot believe how much weight is placed in a glorified internet personality test. We've spent 5 years learning how to practise medicine, how about placing more weight on that? It's a complete joke."**

**"The decision to weight this exam as heavily in the foundation programme application process as a 4–5 year degree plus an additional PhD plus any presentations of publications one may have done is an idiotic error of judgement in itself."**

– Anonymous medical students, in a survey about perceptions of the SJT

Unfortunately, however, this is all a moot point. Because you are stuck with the SJT for the foreseeable future – I desperately wish you weren't, but you are – so there really is no choice but to stay calm, take a deep breath, pop a lorazepam and get on with it. Channel your anger into working hard and efficiently on it, be smart about your strategy and use of resources, then do your absolute best to smash it. Once it's over, you can complain about it to your heart's content, or put it out of your mind and never speak of it again. Or whinge about it in a book as a form of catharsis – that worked for me!

7 *British Journal of Hospital Medicine*, 2015;76:234-8..

## 5.5.7 Summary

In this section, we have looked at what to expect from the Situational Judgement Test in final year. The key points are:

- The SJT is a national, paper-based exam testing you on professionalism, ethics and law. It assesses how you should behave in certain workplace situations.

- There are two sections: ranking questions and MCQs.

- It's worth a wildly disproportionate amount of marks on your Foundation Programme application and can therefore have a big impact on your life and career.

- Ignore anyone who tells you you can't prepare for it: you absolutely **must** prepare for it! Around 4–6 weeks should be enough preparation time.

- Official practice papers and GMC guidance are your most valuable and trustworthy resource: spend the bulk of your time on these and use them to develop general principles about how they want you to behave in certain situations.

- Focus on improving your marks in the corridor of uncertainty: the grey zone between the obviously right and obviously wrong answers.

- Use unofficial resources for quantity – but don't get annoyed when you get their questions 'wrong'. Explanations are subjective and non-official sources therefore can't be trusted.

- Be aware of time pressure and consider doing part two before part one.

- It's natural to get irritated by the SJT but you are stuck with it, so don't let yourself get sidetracked by these feelings – just do the absolute best you can then draw a line under it and move on.

# 5.6 Prescribing Safety Assessment (PSA)

### 5.6.1 What's it all about?

Introduced in 2014, the Prescribing Safety Assessment (PSA) is another national exam, usually taken in final year, which you will need to pass at some point in order to qualify for year 2 of the Foundation Programme. It's not to be confused with the other PSA – prostate-specific antigen – which can also be associated with a pain in the bum.

This PSA lasts for two hours and is all about drugs and prescribing. It's a pass/fail situation, so although you will be given a specific mark this doesn't actually matter much provided you pass (as opposed to the SJT where every extra mark will increase your chances of getting the jobs you want). Nonetheless it's still worth aiming as high as possible to give yourself a healthy margin for error should things go belly up on the day. You'll also want to score highly if you're gunning for prizes at medical school or are aiming for a career in clinical pharmacology and therapeutics.

It goes without saying that no one likes having to do more exams, so you probably ain't too thrilled about this one. Nor was I. However, the good thing about the PSA is it's actually pretty straightforward to prepare for and doesn't require huge amounts of time or wads of cash spent on books and revision courses. Also, to be fair to the people who set it, the content is very reasonable: prescribing is a massive part of being an FY1 so of all the things to examine us on, I really don't begrudge this one!

As we'll see, the main challenges are timekeeping and the technical aspects of the test, rather than the knowledge itself. And these are things which you can quickly get up to speed on with just a little practice. So I wouldn't worry about the PSA because it really is very manageable, and significantly less stressful than the SJT. You've already come through worse, believe me!

### 5.6.2 What does it look like?

The PSA takes place at your medical school across a few different dates in final year (your school will allocate you a particular slot). Some have made it a mandatory part of their medical degree programmes so that you'll have to pass the PSA in order to graduate. Others make you do it just as a formative assessment. Check carefully so that you know exactly what you're up against. Either way, you'll definitely need to sit it before entering the Foundation Programme. If you pass first time, great! If you don't pass on the first try, you can still resit it twice during FY1. However, you will need to pass one of these in order to progress on to FY2. See the website for more information, including the FAQs section under 'resources': www.prescribingsafetyassessment.ac.uk.

The exam itself is fully computer based, with access to the electronic edition of the **BNF** and **BNFc** to look things up. You may also have access to a paper copy of the **BNF** but I would strongly advise you not to use it, for reasons we'll see shortly. There are 200 marks available in total, spread across 60 different questions in eight sections. But not every question is worth the same amount: 'Prescribing' questions are worth ten marks each, 'Prescription Reviews' are worth four and all the others are worth two each; see **Table 5.2** for the full breakdown.

**Table 5.2: The different sections and marks breakdown of the PSA.** Also included is my preferred order for the different sections, but you should devise your own based on your strengths and weaknesses (see **Section 5.6.4**).

| Section | Number of questions | Marks per question | Total marks for the section | My preferred order |
|---|---|---|---|---|
| 1. Prescribing | 8 | 10 | 80 | 1 |
| 2. Prescription review | 8 | 4 | 32 | 2 |
| 3. Planning management | 8 | 2 | 16 | 4 |
| 4. Providing information | 6 | 2 | 12 | 8 |
| 5. Calculation skills | 8 | 2 | 16 | 3 |
| 6. Adverse drug reactions | 8 | 2 | 16 | 7 |
| 7. Drug monitoring | 8 | 2 | 16 | 5 |
| 8. Data interpretation | 6 | 2 | 12 | 6 |
| | Total: 60 questions | | Total: 200 marks | |

## 5.6.3 How to prepare

Doing well in the PSA requires a two-pronged approach. The first prong is your pharmacology knowledge and the second is your specific techniques for the exam itself (particularly your ability to use the Ctrl + F function). Both are important.

Hopefully by now your pharmacology knowledge is already decent and nearly good enough for finals, in which case it will definitely be good enough for the PSA. There are just a few specific things I'd suggest you brush up on as part of your preparation (see **Box 5.10** and **Section 4.4**) as these tend to come up fairly regularly, but otherwise your existing knowledge should be fine. The PSA is part of the reason I've been banging on about pharmacology since **Chapter 3**, because I wanted you to build up this knowledge gradually throughout medical school instead of trying to cram it at the last minute. It's just too big a topic for that and nobody needs that added stress. Maybe you got a little bored of me along the way (no offence taken), but hopefully you took on at least some of my advice to prioritise pharmacology as a subject because this will really start to pay off now. And if you still haven't got around to it, then set some serious time aside and pop back to the pharmacology sections of **Chapters 3** and **4** for pointers. Without knowledge, you will have to look everything up throughout the exam which will *really* slow you down.

| **Important pharmacology topics to brush up on before the PSA** |
| :--- |
| • 'High-risk' drugs: insulin, opioids, steroids, anticoagulants, antibiotics and psychotropics |
| • Prescribing restrictions in pregnancy, breastfeeding, renal impairment and hepatic impairment |
| • Drugs that require therapeutic monitoring, notably gentamicin, amikacin, digoxin and lithium |
| • Analgesics |
| • Fluid and blood product prescribing |
| • Cytochrome P450 enzyme inducer and inhibitors |
| • Converting percentage solutions into dosages and vice versa (remember that a 1% solution contains 1 g per 100 ml). |

Onto prong two then: the specific techniques needed for the exam itself. This is where you will need to put in a bit of legwork to make sure you are completely comfortable with the format and can boss your way through the practice papers at speed. See **Table 5.3** for a list of resources which should be more than enough for your needs. Your medical school will probably also run some sessions – do actually show up to these!

**Start by spending some time on the PSA website and doing the official online practice exams as early as you can. This is by far the best way to get used to the look and feel of the exam and understand what the different sections entail.**

This will also give you a feel for the time pressure under which you will need to finish. Furthermore, like the SJT, the official practice papers are the only source you can truly trust, so personally I relied most heavily on them. The other websites and books are useful for blitzing through a larger volume of practice questions to rehearse your knowledge and improve your speed, but ultimately you will need to take the content with a pinch of salt as it's not provided by the people who write the actual exam. This is less of an issue than with the SJT because pharmacology is much less subjective than ethics and professionalism, but still something to bear in mind!

Some other important things to consider during your practice:

- You may have a choice whether to use the online or print edition of the **BNF**. IMHO you'd be crazy to use print: it's much slower for finding things and the information is potentially out of date if you haven't got the latest edition. Make an early decision to go paperless and don't look back.

- Online access to the **BNF** within the exam is provided through two different portals: NICE and Medicines Complete. They contain the same information, just with a slightly different look and feel to them. Personally I preferred the NICE version, but it really doesn't matter which you use. Try them both out to start with, then just pick your favourite one and stick to it throughout your practice so you get rapid at finding the information you need. You can waste vital minutes on the day if you're faffing around flicking between the two.

- Once you've picked one of these portals, really work on your skills for searching and retrieving information quickly. Ctrl + F is your new best friend: this function lets you search for specific text and find it instantaneously, which is extremely helpful when searching through the long lists of side-effects that accompany every drug. For example, the question might ask which of five medications is most likely to cause dry mouth. You just need to flick back to the **BNF** then Ctrl + F 'dry mouth' within each medication's side-effects page and you'll have an answer in about 30 seconds. The University of Bristol has a useful webpage (https://bristel.cfme.org.uk/tel-guidance/psa/#3) with other helpful keyboard shortcuts.

- Figure out which sections you are weakest on and spend more time practising them. 'Calculation skills' is one that many people find tricky, but also one at which you can get better and faster by putting in some practice. Calculation questions aren't guessable like some of the other sections, so there's a lot to be gained by working on this section in particular. Incorporate your strengths and weaknesses into your exam strategy (**Section 5.6.4**).

- Don't peak too early: to each their own, but personally I wouldn't advise starting your PSA practice more than a month or two before the exam. It doesn't take long to learn the specific techniques, so I preferred to skill myself up in a quick, intensive burst then strike while the iron's hot. By dragging it out over a longer period you may get bored and lose interest, then underperform on the day.

- Redo all the practice papers under strict timed conditions in the last few days before the exam. Even if you remember some of the answers from last time you did them, make sure you still look things up in the **BNF** to make it realistic. Hopefully your times and scores will have improved since the first time you did them.

**Table 5.3: Key resources for the PSA**

| Official practice papers | Available from: www.prescribingsafetyassessment.ac.uk |
|---|---|
| Books | • *Pass the PSA* <br> • *Student Success in the Prescribing Safety Assessment (PSA)* <br> • *Get Ahead! The Prescribing Safety Assessment* |
| Websites | • https://bristel.cfme.org.uk/tel-guidance/psa/#3 <br> • www.prepareforthepsa.com <br> • www.icsmsu.com/exec/education/psa/ |
| Online question banks | • PassMedicine <br> • PasTest <br> • OnExamination |

## 5.6.4  PSA strategy

You're free to skip between the different sections during the exam, which gives you flexibility and allows you to be strategic in your approach. Have a think about this during your practice runs so you can come up with a personalised order that works well for you. You may decide to just run through the sections from start to finish, which is absolutely fine, but don't just do that by default without giving it some thought first.

Keep in mind the marks value of each section as you devise your own strategy. The goals are to maximise your marks, account for your own strengths and weaknesses, and ensure you finish on time. Try to spend the most time on high-yield questions and weak areas where you need to look things up, versus the least time on low-yield questions and areas where you can confidently answer from your own knowledge. I gave you my preferred order in **Table 5.3**, which I'll talk you through shortly. But this is just personal choice – you should come up with your own rather than just following mine! Do this in good time and apply it to your practice run-throughs so you are comfortable with it and won't confuse yourself on the day.

> Consider rearranging the order in which you work through the PSA in order to maximise marks and play to your strengths and weaknesses. You should probably do sections 1 and 2 first as they carry by far the most marks, then do your weakest and most time-consuming sections next so you can spend more time on them and look things up in the *BNF*. Leave your strongest sections till last so you can accelerate towards the finish if time is running short, safe in the knowledge that you can answer quickly and confidently without looking things up.

The first section – 'Prescribing' – is by far the most valuable, with a total of 80 marks. So you should **definitely** spend more time on this section than the others, and to me it makes sense to do it first while you are freshest. Each of these questions includes two marks just for putting in the correct date and signing your name: these are absolute giveaways so make sure you pick them all up!

Personally I'd suggest doing 'Prescription Review' second because with 32 marks, this offers the second most valuable return. I then went to 'Calculation Skills' third because the questions require more time investment and brainpower than other sections, and the answers are free text so you won't really be able to guess them if time is running out. With these three sections done, you've already covered 128 out of 200 marks (64%) so you're absolutely flying.

The order of the other sections is just a matter of personal taste as the questions are all two-mark MCQs and therefore equally valuable. The main issue is how much stuff you need to look up in the **BNF**, because this potentially slows you down compared to questions where you instinctively know the answer. I found that 'Planning Management', 'Drug Monitoring' and 'Data Interpretation' were the most **BNF**-heavy, so I did them next to get them out of the way. Then I finished on 'Adverse Drug Reactions' and 'Providing Information' as these were my strongest areas knowledge-wise so I was able to quickly whip through them without looking too much up and to make educated guesses where required. This is the position you want to be in as the clock is ticking down, not frantically doing calculations or blindly guessing at things you have no idea about.

A final word of warning: it doesn't matter how comfortably you are completing the exams in practice mode, time will **always** be much tighter on the day so please don't get complacent. I finished all my practice papers in good time but then our exam had some mega-tricky prescribing questions which slowed me right down at the beginning. I ended up accelerating into the final two sections, making several educated guesses and finishing with about five seconds to spare. But I did well because I had a good strategy: looking at my breakdown, I did drop marks towards the end but it didn't matter in the slightest because I'd already nailed the earlier parts, despite them taking longer than I wanted, picking up 125 out of 128 marks in the first three sections, for 62.5% of the total. The pass mark in my year was 61% so although I didn't realise it at the time, I had already passed by this point and could have afforded to get every other question wrong! With a strong strategy and some smart, focused preparation, I have every confidence that you can do this too.

### 5.6.5 Summary

In this section, we have looked at what to expect from the Prescribing Safety Assessment in final year. The key points are:

- The PSA is a national, computer-based exam testing you on pharmacology and prescribing.
- It's two hours long, comprising 60 questions across eight sections.
- Some medical schools won't let you graduate without passing it, but for others you have until the end of FY1 if you don't pass it first time.
- Different sections are worth different amounts of marks – it's essential to familiarise yourself with the breakdown.
- Your existing pharmacology knowledge should be good enough, but it's always worth brushing up.
- Focus on your techniques for the exam itself, particularly rapid searching in the electronic **BNF**.
- Use the official practice exams as your main study resource.
- Rearrange the sections into an order that will maximise your scores under time pressure.

# 5.7 Electives

Your elective is a brilliant way to finish medical school, reward yourself for all your hard work and ensure you go out on a high. Electives are essentially a free-choice option to do whatever you want, anywhere in the world, provided it has something to with medicine. Anything you can imagine, medical students have almost certainly done before: space medicine at NASA, canoeing down the Amazon in Peru and learning about dive medicine at the Great Barrier Reef, to name but three examples.

Electives usually last around four to eight weeks and have fairly minimal sign-off requirements, such as writing a short report and getting some basic paperwork signed by your hosts. They've been a tradition and rite of passage for students since the 1970s, and have the potential to be an inspirational and unforgettable highlight of medical school. During the hard times when medical school felt like a long and arduous slog, I found it helpful to visualise my elective as the promised land to look forward to at the end, which kept me going (**Figure 5.7**). And it certainly didn't disappoint when I got there – I spent five weeks in Mauritius on a paediatrics placement at a big national hospital. I learned a lot, experienced a completely different version of medicine and was only expected to attend for a couple of hours each morning, so spent most of my time lying on the beach with my wife and kids. It was absolute bliss, let me tell you!

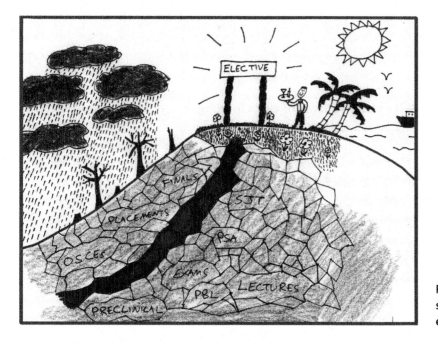

Figure 5.7: The sunny uplands of the elective!

There is a lot of advice out there on how to plan your elective (see **Box 5.11**) so we'll stick to the essentials. Here are my top tips to help you with your planning:

1. **Decide exactly what you want to get out of it.** This is the most important question, and everything else should start to fall into place once you've got the answer. For me, it was clear: I wanted somewhere hot and sunny that I could relax and recharge before FY1, with the added bonus of experiencing medicine in a very different healthcare system to the UK. Others want to boost their surgical skills, do some research, get experience at a particular institution, go travelling or visit friends and family abroad. Whatever your motivation: keep it in focus as this will really help you with your planning, which can easily get overwhelming if you don't have a clear objective in mind.

2. **Don't feel you have to go abroad.** Loads of students stay in the UK for their electives, for a wide variety of reasons. You can still do something totally new and exciting and have an amazing experience, so don't let anyone else (or their social media feed) make you feel like you have to get on a plane for your elective to be worthwhile. You can also do a mix: if your budget only stretches to two weeks abroad, for example, you could top that up with an additional four-week placement at home to meet your university's requirements.

3. **Consider whether to do a 'package' trip or organise it yourself.** If you are going abroad, agencies such as Work the World provide elective placements in a wide range of exotic locations. This can take a lot of the hassle and risk out of organising it, but is usually more expensive. At the time of writing, packages ranged from £1040 for two weeks in Nepal to £2390 for six weeks in Tanzania.

4. **Look for sources of extra funding.** Budget is of course a major consideration for most students, but help is available so don't just assume that you won't be able to afford what you want. Check out the helpful articles from the **Student BMJ** and Royal Medical Benevolent Fund in **Box 5.11**, and ask your medical school about the various bursaries, grants and awards available. Be aware that you will need to apply early for these – often at least a year in advance.

5. **Do your research.** Once you are narrowing in on potential destinations, make sure to read reviews on sites like the Electives Network and speak to students who've done that placement before. Try to find out what the day-to-day schedule is like and what their expectations are for your attendance. If these don't align with your

overarching goals, then you should probably rethink before you commit. Other important things to research include transport, accommodation, weather, the local culture, vaccinations, travel insurance and indemnity, visas and any other extra costs once you arrive.

6. **Make the most of it.** Whatever your ideas and expectations for your elective, remember that you probably won't get many opportunities like this again once you embark on your career as a doctor. It's completely up to you how you use it, but don't let apathy, disorganisation or laziness dictate your plans because you will almost certainly regret it later. Trust me, having just finished an exhausting stretch of 12-hour days on the medical admissions team in an extremely busy London hospital, confronting stress, deaths and numerous PR examinations, I would be back on that plane to Mauritius in a heartbeat!

---

**Useful resources for planning your elective:**   **Box 5.11**

- The BMA has absolutely tons of useful guidance, including case studies, budgeting tips and a checklist for your planning: www.bma.org.uk/advice/career/going-abroad/medical-electives
- The Electives Network has thousands of reviews by previous students, and is an essential port of call if you are planning your own trip abroad:www.electives.net/
- Work the World offers a range of elective packages in Africa, Asia and Latin America, which is great if you don't want the hassle of organising everything yourself: www.worktheworld.co.uk/medical-electives
- The Adventure Medic has loads of great ideas, articles and testimonials if you're looking for an 'adventurous' type of elective: www.theadventuremedic.com/category/electives/
- The Royal Medical Benevolent Fund has more advice on funding your elective: https://rmbf.org/medical-students/sources-of-funding-for-your-elective/
- The *BMJ* has many helpful articles about planning and maximising your elective, including this one about funding: www.bmj.com/content/343/sbmj.d5851. You can find others (including one I wrote!) by searching on their homepage
- Read some of the debate around so-called 'medical voluntourism', i.e. how much host countries really benefit from the presence of western medical students. This is worth pondering if you are going to a developing country. This article from *Huffington Post* is a good place to start: www.bit.ly/Box5-11

# 5.8 Congratulations!

Congratulations on reaching the end of medical school! It's an even bigger achievement than getting in, and you should be extremely proud of yourself. This point marks the end of our journey together. I hope you have found my advice helpful and enjoyed your studies as much as I did. Let me know what you think by tweeting @davidbrill. I'd love to hear from you!

Whatever happens, please don't forget how far you've come since you first applied to medical school: you are now about to be a qualified doctor yourself, no matter how unbelievable that may seem! Remember what it felt like to be a wide-eyed newbie, and don't take for granted how much you have to offer to students in the years below. You are now an expert in their eyes and they are looking up to you: please encourage them, support them, help them and be a good role model for them. The future of our profession may depend on it.

Medical school might have seemed hard, but in many ways the really hard part starts now. Becoming an FY1 is in equal measures exciting and terrifying, but I can assure you it does get easier with time and you might even start to find it enjoyable! Be organised, be helpful, be proactive and be efficient. Work within your competencies and ask a senior if you are feeling out of your depth. Remember the time management and coping skills we have discussed throughout this book, and you will be absolutely fine. **You've got this.** I know you have.

# Index